The Radia

Once the Radiants get our bodies, they're supposed to move them to someplace on the other side of the world, where there's less chance of encountering people who knew the bodies in life.

Most of the Radiants we have in Sparrow Creek look like they come from East India, the rules about relocation being what they are. They have their own enclave on the far side of the creek, away from the rest of town. They do some mixing, though not a whole lot. You see them in the Quick Lunch Diner and at the library and hanging around the bus station. Sometimes they're at the public pool in the summer—guess they get hot same as we do—but when they get into the pool, most regular people get out.

I don't know. There's just something creepy about swimming with corpses.

—from "Radiance," Nina Kiriki Hoffman

Whitley Strieber's *Aliens*

The Horror Writers Association presents

WHITLEY STRIEBER'S

ALIENS

Edited by Whitley Strieber

POCKET STAR BOOKS

New York London Toronto Sydney Tokyo Singapore

This book consists of works of fiction. Names, characters, places and incidents are products of the authors' imaginations or are used fictitiously. Any resemblance to actual events or locales or persons living or dead is entirely coincidental.

An *Original* Publication of POCKET BOOKS

A Pocket Star Book published by
POCKET BOOKS, a division of Simon & Schuster Inc.
1230 Avenue of the Americas, New York, NY 10020

ISBN: 0-671-88597-9

First Pocket Books printing January 1999

10 9 8 7 6 5 4 3 2 1

Cover art by John Stephens

Printed in the U.S.A.

Copyright Notices

Acknowledgments

I would like to thank all the authors who submitted for this collection. Choosing was agony, because so many of the stories were so good. Without the thoughtful and well-informed editorial contribution and support of Anne Strieber, this volume would not have been possible.

—Whitley Strieber

CONTENTS

INTRODUCTION

Aliens. Are they here? Well, nobody's landed on the White House lawn yet, but we're starting to consider the possibility.

But if they landed, if they were here, what would it be like? We can't know that for certain—which is, at the moment, a big part of the fun, because there's room to dream, to wonder . . . and to worry.

What if, for example, they were like some of the aliens in these stories? Now, that would be interesting.

Or—perhaps not. Maybe it would be best if we didn't go down where Buddy lives in Gary Braunbeck's "In Hollow Houses." Then again, it's a journey too interesting to miss. Or perhaps getting involved with the Radiants in Nina Hoffman's "Radiance" would not be such a good idea. Except that it's so-o-o tempting.

These stories aren't based on real close-encounter cases, but on the human imagination as it probes the darkness of a relationship that may or may not be happening. In a sense, this is the best of all times to write fiction about this subject, precisely because we know so little about what's going on.

Who's to say there are no Travelers like the ones in Adam-Troy Castro's "Fuel," a web of creatures from across the whole of space-time, each a fugitive from a different type of alien existence, or that Tracy Knight's "Glassy Apes" aren't waiting outside all the windows of the world?

All of these stories have one thing in common: they are speculations about the nature and motives of alien life-forms. All are animated by the notion that such life-forms will be extremely strange, that they will challenge the limits of meaning and make the surreal seem comfortable and familiar.

I suspect that the imaginary aliens in this collection may actually be as strange as the real thing. At least, some of the stories certainly capture the aggressively bizarre flavor of the real close-encounter experience, even if they don't mirror its reported structure.

The interesting thing about this quantum machine that we call the human imagination is that it bears a relationship to reality that we really do not understand. We do not know the degree to which the mind creates reality, and therefore cannot know whether or not the stories we are writing in the present are simply stories, or the secret architecture of the future.

Which gets me to "Jolene's Motel," a place that

you and I had both better hope isn't in our futures. And yet, going there with Esther Friesner and her characters is wonderfully eerie fun. Certainly, it couldn't really happen. Unless—is the human mind the weaver of reality? Oh, I hope not, because if it is, we need to have a word with Esther, folks. We need a little more information about that weapon, you see . . .

All of these stories have the power to send a chill down the spine. In fact, to send it plummeting toward absolute zero. Actually, can you go colder than that?

To a person like me, who has seen firsthand how plastic reality is, stories such as these possess a very special sort of a bite. Every time I read a story of this type, I find myself wondering if the author isn't in some way connected to the close-encounter experience, if it isn't buried somewhere in his or her life.

One of the ways that people deal with a close encounter is through sublimation. To give one example, there is a witness who had an implant removed from his leg that he believes was put in by aliens who abducted him along with his brother. This is an especially interesting case, because the implant has received a substantial amount of scientific study and has a very bizarre chemical composition that may even include an as-yet-undiscovered isotope of sulfur. While he recalls the experience and acknowledges it, his brother does not.

Instead, what his brother has done has been to build his home in the shape of a UFO and spend a good deal of time thinking and talking about aliens—all without looking directly at his own past. If he was a writer, he might very possibly have created a story much like any one of these.

So, what really lies behind this fascinating collection of speculations? Could it be that the shadow behind the shadow is real?

What might it mean, then, that this collection of delicious terrors would be inspired by the possibility that their authors are victims of alien abduction and that they have repressed their experience? I'm not trying to scare you (too much), but there is always the possibility that some of this stuff is *true*.

So now I've said it. We've always said that the encounter experience would be extremely strange. Okay, then, some of the encounters you are going to have between these pages are going to fulfill that defintion, in spades. Now, I wouldn't maintain that any of this stuff is going to happen. Of course not.

I know that I shouldn't say this. Maybe it's even a little dangerous to say it. But what if some of it *is* going to happen?

My God, what if it already has?

—Whitley Strieber

WHITLEY STRIEBER'S

ALIENS

IN HOLLOW HOUSES

Gary A. Braunbeck

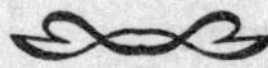

Still there are moments when one feels free from one's own identification with human limitations and inadequacies. At such moments, one imagines that one stands on some small spot on an unknown planet, gazing in amazement at the cold yet profoundly moving beauty of the eternal, the unfathomable: life and death flow into one, and there is neither evolution nor destiny; only being.

—Albert Einstein

Heaven wheels above you displaying to you her eternal glories and still your eyes are on the ground.

—Dante

I

Down in the Rusty Room where Buddy lived these words had been written on one of the walls:

someone come
i'm tired of naming things
and then forgetting their names
the voice in the sky is
loneliness
and the night is
restlessness

someone come

Even though she was only a little girl of six (well, *almost* six), she knew that Buddy had written the words, and that it was some kind of prayer, and that made her sad because she knew what it was like to feel so scared and tired and alone, like you belonged somewhere else but there wasn't anybody listening to you when you asked to leave.

and where do I live?
under the tracks of the el
in a cardboard box
that's falling apart

within the cell life is hard, life is long
within the cell, life is hard

someone please come

II

Leah watched in silence as her mother handed the baby over to the man in the dark coat and knew she wouldn't be seeing her little sister again. It always happened this way: Mommy would go away with the men in the dark coats to the Shiny Place (that's what Mommy called it) and Leah would be all by herself for weeks at a time in the abandoned warehouse that was her home; it was kind of scary for a little while after Mommy left, but it was easier getting the people at the restaurants to give her food when she was by herself—"Oh, you poor child," they all said, stuffing bread and hamburgers and doughnuts and little cartons of milk into the paper bags, "What kind of a mother would do this to a child?"—so she never had to dig through the garbage Dumpsters like she had to with Mommy. And there was Merc and Chief Wetbrain who were always on their corner a few blocks away; they were really nice and had helped her before . . . but mostly there was Buddy. She thought it was a good thing that she had Buddy around to take care of her when Mommy was gone; he always made things better.

The dark-coat man took the baby, smiled down at it, then snapped his fingers; another man in a dark coat and sunglasses (Leah wondered why none of the dark-coat men ever took their sunglasses off, even at night) got out of the car and handed Mommy a thick envelope. That made Leah feel even worse. She knew there was money in the envelope that the dark-coat man was giving to Mommy for the baby, and Mommy would use it to buy more needle-stuff that would last until the next time the men in the dark coats returned to take her to the Shiny Place, and after a couple of weeks she'd come back all pregnant, then have the baby, then the dark-coat men'd be there with their envelopes full of money.

Leah wanted to cry. She hadn't even got to give her little sister a name—and this had been her *first* sister, too.

She felt a tear forming and closed her eyes, taking a deep breath and Removing herself (that's what Buddy called it) from everything going on around her, watching as silvery shimmer-bursts of light went off behind her closed lids, and she did just as Buddy had taught her, she reached out in her mind like in a daydream and snagged a ride on one of the shimmers—

And saw the Earth and the Moon as they must have looked to astronauts moving through the cold, glittering depths of the cosmos; the dry, pounded surface of the moon, its craters dark and secretive and dead as an old bone; just beyond was a milky-white radiance that cast liquid-gray shadows across the lunarscape while distant stars winked at her, then a burst of heat and pressure and suddenly she was below the moist, gleaming membrane of the bright blue sky, Earth rising exuberantly into her line of sight: she marveled at the majestic, swirling drifts of white clouds covering and uncovering the half-hidden masses of land and watched the continents themselves in motion, drifting apart on their crustal plates, held afloat by the molten fire.

And when the plates had settled and the rivers had carved their paths and the trees had spread their wondrous arms, there came next the People and their races and mysteries through the ages, and in her mind she danced through some of those Mysteries, Buddy holding her hand as they stood atop places with wonderful and odd names, places like Cheop's pyramid and the tower of Ra, Zoroaster's Temple and the Javanese Borobudur, the Krishna shrine, the Valhalla plateau and Woton's Throne, and then they started dancing through King Arthur's castle and Gawain's abyss and Lancelot's point, then they went to Solomon's Temple at Moriah, then the Aztec amphitheatre, Toltec point, Cardenas butte, and Alarcon terrace before stopping at last in front of the great Wall of Skulls at Chicén Itzà: The skulls were awash by a sea of glowing colors, changing shape in the lights from above, their mouths opening as if to speak to her, flesh spreading across bone to form faces and her heart—oh, her heart felt almost freed and—

Mommy smacked her on the shoulder. "Stop daydreaming, damn you."

The dark-coat man handed the baby to one of his friends, then walked over to Leah, took off his sunglasses, and smiled down at her. His eyes were cold and black and made Leah feel like he'd swallow her up if she looked into them for too long.

"Please don't," said Mommy. "She's all I've got."

One of the other men grabbed Leah's mother and held her back.

"All you've got like my ass chews gum," said the dark-coat man. "You have about as much love in your heart for this child as I do for you, you worthless piece of shit."

"Don't you call my mommy names!" shouted Leah.

"I apologize," said the dark-coat man, kneeling down in front of Leah. "Tell me, sweetheart, how old are you now?"

"I'll be six pretty soon."

"The thirteenth of next month, as a matter of fact," he said. "And you know what's going to happen then?"

"Uh-uh."

"Why, we're going to come back and take *both* you and your mommy to a birthday party for you."

"Really? In the Shiny Place?"

The dark-coat man shot an angry glance at Leah's mother. "Chatty little thing, aren't you?"

"Go fuck yourself."

"And charming, to boot." He looked back at Leah. "Yes, sweetheart, we're going to have a birthday party for you in the Shiny Place. Then you and your mommy can live there, if you want. It's very nice; it's clean and you can watch television and play games and there'll be food every day and you won't have to worry about ever being left alone again."

"Can I still see my friends?"

Something in the dark-coat man's eyes brightened when she asked this. "What friends do you mean, sweetheart?"

"You know . . . Merc and Chief Wetbrain, and Long Red—she's a singer who comes around to visit Merc sometimes."

"*Of course* you can still see them, Leah. We'll even bring them to the party if you want."

"Could they live with us, maybe?"

"Maybe. Are there any other friends you want to come to the party?"

She almost told him about Buddy but something in the way he'd said *any other friends* didn't sound very nice, so Leah just shook her head.

The dark-coat man stopped smiling. "Well, then . . . you think about it, sweetheart. If there's anyone else you want to be there, you just tell us where they are and we'll invite them." He reached out and touched her cheek. His hand felt like cold, raw restaurant meat. "Listen, sweetheart, we need to, uh . . . do something to you right now, if it's okay."

"Don't touch her!" shouted Mommy.

"Shut up," said the dark-coat man. Then, to Leah: "Would you do a big favor for me? Would you get into the backseat of my car and let us take a little blood from your arm?"

"W-why?"

"It's all right, Leah; the man who'll do it is a doctor so you don't have to—"

"I don't like needles," said Leah, as much to her mother as the dark-coat man.

"I know you don't, honey, but we need it . . . we need it in case your little sister gets sick, see? You both have the same blood type—do you know what that is?"

"Uh-huh."

"Good. You both have the same blood type, and it's very rare; you're the only other girl in this part of the country who has it, and if something happens and your little sister needs blood, we wouldn't have any."

Leah thought about it for a moment. "Will it hurt?"

"Only a little sting, I promise."

Leah's lower lip trembled. "I don't want her to be sick."

"Oh, she's not sick, hon, but if she *were* to get sick—"

"Okay."

"I won't let you!" shouted Mommy.

"That's enough from you," said the dark-coat man, rising to his feet. "She loves her little sister, don't you, Leah? She only wants to help, and if she doesn't, that might spoil things. We don't want to spoil things for her, *do we?*"

"Will she be there?" asked Leah, pointing at the baby. "At my party?"

"If you want."

"I do, I really do. I never had a little sister before."

"Does she have a name?"

"Uh-uh."

"Ah, well . . . that can be one of your presents. You can give your little sister a name. Would you like that?"

"Oh, *yes!*"

"Consider it done, then."

Leah got into the backseat and let the nice old doctor with the gray hair take some blood from her arm; it took a lot longer than she thought it would because he had to fill a clear plastic bag, and it left her feeling a little dizzy but then he gave her some lemonade and cookies and she felt better.

As she sat there finishing off the cookies and starting in on the King Dons ("Maybe you'd better have something more," the doctor had said), she heard Mommy talking with the dark-coat man.

"What're you going to do with her?" said Mommy.

"None of your business. You've not asked about what happened to any of the others, so why the sudden concern?"

"Because . . . I dunno . . . she's not such a bad kid, y' know? I love—"

"Oh, spare me. God, you're disgusting."

"You can't talk to me like that!"

"I can talk to you any way I damned well please. Aside from the fact it took us three fucking years to find you, the only reason we've let you keep her this long is because she's formed—for whatever bizarre reasons—an emotional attachment to you. *She loves you.* We didn't expect that. But don't think that means you're safe, dearie. You could be disappeared like *that*"—he snapped his fingers—"and no one would give a damn."

"Maybe," said Mommy. "And maybe not. Maybe I got friends around town, you know? And maybe I gave a couple of them copies of a letter I wrote, and they'll send those letters if I turn up missing."

"Do you really think that just because my division works outside the boundaries of the federal government we can't affect something so puny as the U.S. Postal Service? Christ! You don't *deserve* to be her mother."

"What is she to you, anyway?"

"A pinball," said the dark-coat man, then laughed.

"Oh, my, the expression on your face—BoBo the Dog-Faced Boy looked more intelligent. You have no idea what I'm talking about, do you?"

"You never made a whole lot of sense in all the years I've known you."

"And I fear it's prevented us from becoming closer. The heart breaks. Listen: a few weeks ago I was in Jerusalem checking out reports on a little girl who we thought might be like Leah. What happened with her is none of your business and secondary to the point of my story, anyway.

"I was walking through one of the oldest sections of the city and admiring its beauty, when I got to thinking about how Jerusalem was perceived in earlier times: many religious groups considered it—and still *do* consider it—the center of the universe, the navel of the world where heaven and earth join. It was there at the center of the universe that God spoke to His prophets and the People of the Book; Jews come to worship at the wall of their temple near the Holy of Holies, Christians come to follow the steps of their Lord in His Final Passion, and Muslims worship at the Dome of the Rock where Mohammed received the Koran.

"In ancient times, there was a center to the old city marked by Roman crossroads that divided the city and the earth into four quadrants—the fulcrum of medieval geography. Most of the roads disappeared long ago, but to this day, at each corner of the crossroads, there still stands a Roman pillar. So I found myself wandering into the very center-within-the-center of the universe. Do you know what's there? Of all the shrines and statues, temples and rocks, symbols and what-have-you that *could* be there to mark the exact, precise center of the universe, can you guess what I found?

"A pinball parlor. Rows and rows of pinball machines. Astonishing. I laughed, I couldn't help it. Determinists think of the universe as a clockwork device. I see it as a pinball machine. Playing pinball requires total concentration, the right combination of skill and chance, an understanding and mastery of indeterminacy as the balls fly about, interacting with the bumpers and cushions. It creates an ersatz reality that integrates into the human nervous system in a remarkable way, and I realized that it was no accident that pinball machines stand at the center of the universe, because in order to know the universe we must observe it, and in the act of observation, uncontrolled and random processes are initiated into reality. I can see from that blank look in your eyes that I'm losing you, so I'll make it simple: children like your daughter will someday soon become the pinballs in the machine of the universe, and whoever has them, whoever controls them, is master of the game and need not worry that the device will tilt on them."

"Man, you are *so* full of shit."

"I take back what I said about you before; you don't disgust me. I pity you too much to feel disgust."

"Feeling better now?" asked the doctor, jostling Leah's arm.

"Yes, sir," she said. "Thanks for the King Dons. I don't get to have a lot of snacks."

"Would you like some more to take with you?"

"Yes, please."

As the doctor was putting the extra packs of King Dons into a paper bag for her, he asked, "Tell me, Leah, do you get many headaches?"

"Sometimes."

"Are they bad?"

"Yeah. Sometimes they hurt *real* bad."

"Can you show me where they start, these headaches?"

"Sure." She put a finger on the bridge of her nose. "Right here. I get a runny nose, too. Sometimes my nose bleeds a little."

"I see," said the doctor, then reached into one of his pockets and pulled out a bottle of pills. "What you've got, Leah, is a condition called sinusitis. It's not uncommon for children of . . . for children like yourself. Don't you worry yourself, hon; it's not too serious, if treated properly. Here, you take these pills—and *don't* let your mommy see them, all right? She'd only take them away from you."

" 'Kay . . . ?"

"The red ones are for your headaches, all right? Take one when the pain gets real bad. The blue ones are for infection; you should take one of those three times a day. Can you remember all that, Leah?"

"Yes, sir."

The doctor smiled and touched her face; his hand wasn't at all like the dark-coat man's; his hand was warm and kind, like a Grandpa's hand—or, rather, how Leah *imagined* a Grandpa's hand would feel.

"You're a very pretty little girl, Leah, has anyone told you that?"

"No, sir."

"And with the 'sir'! So polite."

"Thank you."

"I know a lot of this must be confusing for you, dear, but when we come back and take you to your birthday party next month, you'll understand everything."

"My little sister's gonna be there. The other man said so."

"And so she shall be." Then the doctor leaned forward, pulled Leah close, and whispered, "Your brothers might be there, as well."

Leah felt her heart skip a beat. "All of them?"

"Yes. And maybe—and you must not tell this to *anyone*—maybe your daddy will be there, too."

Leah was so excited she could barely contain herself. For all of her life she'd wondered about her daddy; who he was, where he came from, what he did for a living. All she really knew was that the men drove Mommy to see Daddy whenever they took her away. And now she might maybe get to see her daddy for the first time.

In her heart, wizards, angels, and faeries danced.

"Oh, *thank you,*" she said, then gave the doctor a great big hug and kissed him on the cheek. He hugged her back, and there was something sad in the way he did it, something that made Leah think of the words on Buddy's wall: *the voice in the night sky is loneliness . . .*

"You remember about the pills," said the doctor, "and about our little secret about your daddy, okay?"

"Okay," said Leah, stuffing the bottle of pills into

one of her pockets and climbing out of the car, the bag of King Dons clutched to her chest like discovered treasure. She wondered if Buddy liked King Dons, if he'd ever had them, and looked forward to sharing them with her best-best friend in the whole world.

Mommy grabbed Leah's arm and they ran out of the alley. The only sound Leah could hear now was the laughter of the dark-coat man; it bounced off the alley walls, ugly and mean, coming after her and Mommy like some crazy junkyard dog. The sound wailed and roared in the slick darkness of the rain-dampened streets, and under the laughter Leah could hear her little sister starting to cry and suddenly she felt awful, like she'd just run over a bird with her bike. She felt like a killer. She didn't want to leave her sister in the alley with the dark-coat man. The alley was cold and wet and dark and smelled like somebody threw up.

"Mommy, please go and get her back."

"Be quiet."

"Please? She's c-c-crying, hear? She misses us and—"

"I said shut up!" screamed her mother, slapping Leah hard across the face. "Shut your miserable little mouth, goddammit, or I swear I'll . . . I'll let Jewel take you up to his room next time!"

Leah went rigid with fear. Jewel was the short little bald-headed man Mommy bought her needle-stuff from. He was old and wrinkly and sweated all the time and was always trying to touch Leah whenever he saw her. "Young and tasty," he said. "I like 'em when they're young and tasty." Leah didn't know what Jewel wanted to do with her, but she knew it probably wasn't very nice because Jewel had a little girl named Denise who was with him all the time, and she always had bruises and cuts on her face and over her body and sometimes burn marks around her wrists and she never said anything whenever Leah talked to her and her eyes were always staring out at something only she seemed able to see, and whatever it was she saw made her empty.

"Oh, no, *please Mommy, d-d-don't do that!*"

"Then be quiet. You've caused me enough trouble as it is."

Leah's face twisted into a tight, hard, painful knot, and she couldn't stop the tears from coming then. She thought that her mommy loved her and would never do something like that. But maybe—

You have about as much love in your heart for that child as I do for you . . .

Mommy only said that because of how she felt about the baby. Leah hoped so but she couldn't ask her mother because Mommy would only get madder, so she decided to wait and tell Buddy about it tonight after Mommy did her needle-thing and rolled her eyes and shook and fell asleep sort-of. Buddy would say the right things to make her understand and make it all better.

Leah was glad that Mommy didn't know about Buddy and his secret Rusty Room underneath the warehouse basement.

Buddy didn't like her mother. Not one little bit.

III

and where do i live?
in the alleys behind the
cans
abandonment my blanket
no way to slough the fever
and where do i live?
in songs unheard
in the flutter of bound wings that
don't know they're bound
where?
somewhere else
not here

within the cell, life is long, life is hard,
within the cell, life is hard

who will take me?

IV

Leah smiled as Chief Wetbrain drew a chalk circle around him, scooted into its center (he had to scoot everywhere because he didn't have any legs), and started playing his saxophone. Leah thought it was too bad that people called him Chief Wetbrain (she did it, too, and always felt bad afterward) because it was such an ugly name and they only used it because he got drunk a lot on account of the pain in his leg stumps. His real name was Jimmy NightEagle, and

Leah wished he'd tell more people to call him that; it was the name of a king, and that's what Jimmy was in her eyes.

Mommy was down the street at Jewel's apartment buying her needle-stuff and had said it was okay for Leah to go visit with her friends. Leah liked listening to Jimmy play his saxophone; his music made her feel less scared and sometimes, if she closed her eyes and listened real hard, the way Buddy had taught her, she could hear the unspoken words in Jimmy's songs: *Who will take me? I don't belong here.*

(. . . someone come . . .)

Listening the way Buddy had taught her, she heard Jimmy's song cry out a tale composed of notes that became Kachinas and Crow Mothers and They Who Breathed the Land into Being; she heard it turn round in the breeze and catch raindrops that held his memories of nights on the plains, soaring above the heads of the people as they passed, sprinkling them with hints of things he still knew and they had long ago forgotten, secrets of the Earth and Time hidden in the silences between the notes; a breath, a beat, songs of the Elders and their tales of the Fiery-Sky Ones, another breath, another beat, and the notes multiplied like the birds of the sky after solstice, power, strength, and courage in his grip as he pulled the sax closer to his ruined body, breathing his soul into the reeds like a fine medicine man should—and over there, a glint in a passing pair of eyes, yes, as the song banked on the winds and came back to him, more than it was before, making him feel that he was back among his people again, back where he should have been all along, grace covering him like tree-fallen leaves in autumn, so good, yes, I am ready: the time is upon me to fly.

Jimmy stopped playing as a young man in a three-piece suit walked by and threw some change into a tin cup sitting between his stumps. Jimmy smiled and lifted his hat to the young man in thanks, then looked into the cup. "*Sokelas!*" he said, taking out the three quarters and jingling them in his hand. "And my folks used to worry about me making a living as a jazz musician." He looked at Leah, then gave her one of the coins. "That's just for being a pretty sight to these tired eyes."

"How come you're tired?"

"How come I'm—? I'm sorry, I didn't mean to snap like that."

"'S okay."

"No, it isn't," said Jimmy, taking hold of her hand. "I'm tired because I've been having too many bad dreams lately. I'm tired because I feel more and more like *eceyanunia*—a fool—every day. I'm tired because no one answers the music." He pulled her a little closer, putting his arm around her waist. Leah liked it when Jimmy hugged her, it wasn't at all like when Jewel touched her—moist and chilly and sick-making; Jimmy's hugs were gentle and kind and made her feel loved.

"There was a time, Leah, before I left to be educated in the white schools, when I would play my music at night under the stars and know that it would be heard by *Matotipila,* would linger in the heart of *Wanagitacanku,* answered by *Tayamni,* but not here, not in the city. There's too much noise, too much anger and violence, and the buildings block out the heavens. Sometimes I find myself wondering if the heavens are still really there." He shook his head. "Does any of this make sense to you?"

"Uh-huh, some."

"I like you very much, Leah. You're a good friend and I will miss you when I'm gone."

"You're not leaving, are you?"

"Oh, not right now, probably not for a while, but I've been thinking about it for a long time. Especially since the dreams started."

"What kind of dreams? What happens in them?"

Jimmy laughed but there was no humor in it. "You see, that's the thing, I can't really say what happens because I don't know, exactly. It's not so much what *happens* in them, anyway, as it is . . . the *impression* they leave when I wake up. I feel like I don't belong here, but I can't go back home because I don't belong there anymore, either. Not that they'd have me, and if they wouldn't, then . . . who *will* take me?" He reached out and massaged one of his stumps. "Get drunk and pass out under a trailer, have it back over you and crush your legs—do this once, and people think you're incompetent."

Leah giggled.

"Ah, good girl," said Jimmy. "There was a time when you wouldn't've realized I was making a joke."

"But it was only a half-joke. It was still funny, though."

"I'm glad you liked it. I like hearing you laugh; it's a lovely sound. I wish you made it more often."

"I know. Buddy says that I—" She gasped, then covered her mouth with her hands, eyes wide. Oh,

God! She'd never mentioned Buddy to anyone before and now . . .

"Buddy," whispered Jimmy. "So that's his name? In my dream he was called *Peye'wik:* It-Is-Approaching."

Slowly, Leah pulled her hands away from her mouth. "You know about Buddy?"

Jimmy reached into one of his pockets and took out a folded piece of paper that he handed to Leah. "There was one image from the dreams that I remembered early on, and I drew it on that paper. Take a look and tell me if those're—tell me if it looks familiar to you."

Leah unfolded the piece of paper. Most of it was blank, except for two large, dark, slanted, opposing almond-shapes in the middle. *"Buddy's eyes,"* she said.

" 'Someone come,' " said Jimmy.

"W-what?"

" 'Someone come.' Buddy wrote those words on a wall somewhere, didn't he?"

"Uh-huh."

"He's very lonely, isn't he, your Buddy?"

"I guess. But with him it's like . . . it's like with Denise, that girl who lives with Jewel?"

Jimmy closed his eyes and nodded his head. *"A Hollow House.* More pain than person. *Goddamn* that little pervert."

"With Buddy, it's like he's so lonely he don't even know it."

"Oh, I doubt that," said Jimmy. "I think he knows exactly how lonely he is. He's just like us, Leah; he should be somewhere else."

Just then Merc came around the corner pulling something behind him that made a funny *thunka-thunka-shisk! thunka-thunka-shisk!* noise: an orange crate nailed to a set of planks that were supported by roller-skate wheels.

"Oh, *man,*" said Merc, coming to a stop next to them. "I read this article in the science section of the paper yesterday about that damn woolly mammoth they found upstate a couple weeks ago—you know, the one that was almost completely preserved? Anyway, these science dudes, they were makin' all this brouhaha over the buttercups that were in the thing's mouth. Seems these buttercups were as totally preserved as the mammoth, right? But what makes everything so righteously fucked—oops, sorry, Leah, gotta learn to watch my mouth—what makes it all really weird, right, is that buttercups evidently release some kind of chemical into your system when you eat them that acts like a natural anti-freeze, y'dig? The mammoth had itself a bellyful of buttercups, so they're saying that's why it was so well-preserved, but—whoa, almost lost track of where I's going with this—but the thing is, buttercups can only grow in a moist, warm climate, like around seventy-eight degrees or so, and these buttercups in the mammoth's belly, they weren't dehydrated, and neither was the mammoth. You know what that means? That means in order for the mammoth to've been preserved so well and without dehydration, the temperature had to've dropped from around eighty degrees to something like three-hundred *below zero* in a matter of seconds! And these science wizards, they got no idea what happened, let alone how it could've happened, and if they can't speculate on what happened, then they got no way of being able to predict if or when it might happen again. Man, I tell you, that *messed up* my breakfast big time! Knowing that at any given second we could all be slammed into the fuc—uh, *friggin'* deep freeze and there's nothing we can do about it. It could all be over"—he snapped his fingers—"like *that*, and I spent ten minutes trying to decide what to wear today. Not that I got what you'd call an *ex-ten-sive* wardrobe. That game on your head, or what?"

"Do you ever just say 'hello'?" asked Jimmy.

"Uh, yeah, right. Forgettin' my manners left and right today. Hello."

"What'cha got there?" said Leah, pointing at the orange crate.

"Huh? Oh, this?" He stood back and gestured with his arms like a model at an automobile show. "This here's the new Chiefmobile, first one off the line."

Jimmy stared. "You . . . you *made* this for me?"

"I get kinda tired of watching you do the Stumpy Dance when you walk. Them little short steps give me a pain. Takes forever to get anywhere with you. I figure this way, you hop in the Chiefmobile and we'll be *burnin'* up pavement. Do wonders for clearing up my schedule. So, you like it?"

Jimmy shrugged (but gave Leah a quick wink), and said, "It's all right, if you like that sort of thing."

"*That sort of thing?* I been digging through dumpsters for the last two weeks trying to find four sets of wheels that're all the same size and all you got to say is, 'If you like that sort of thing'? Talk about your ingrates. Here we got you *trans-por-tation,* Chief. You hear what I'm saying? Take your act on the road. Make 'em big wampum, go truckin' on down that Happy Trail in style."

"It is perhaps one of the ten most wondrous sights I have ever beheld in all my life. Why, in all the history of history itself, there has never been a more resplendent orange-crate chariot. I think I'm safe in saying that, yes."

Merc cocked his head to one side as if trying to decide if Jimmy was yanking his chain or not, then gave a quick nod. "Well, that's more like it. Man needs to know his labors're appreciated."

"Very much," said Jimmy, reaching out and patting the side of Merc's leg. "Very much. Thank you."

Merc knelt down and clapped Jimmy on the shoulder. "No *hombre* of mine's gonna be stumpin' round and giving himself more pain."

The two of them looked at one another for a moment.

In the silence, Leah heard the song of two hearts: friendship.

She ran over and gave Merc a big hug and kiss; she couldn't help it.

"What's that for?" asked Merc.

"'Cause you're a sweetie."

"Uh-oh, this's starting to get too warm and fuzzy for me—but thanks for the hug and smoochie, darlin'. Nice to know the Merc's still got it for the ladies—speaking of: You seen Red around here today, Chief?"

"No, but I heard she's selling—uh, I heard she's *singing* at some club in the East End."

"Singing?" Merc looked from Jimmy to Leah, then

back to Jimmy again. "Oh, yeah, right! I forgot about her, uh, *singing* engagement."

"I know what a hooker is," said Leah. "You don't have to talk around me like I'm stupid or something."

Jimmy and Merc burst out laughing.

"Here I thought we were being so *co-vert,*" said Merc.

"It's okay," said Leah. "I tell everybody that Long Red's a singer so they won't know."

"Well, that's darned thoughtful of you." Merc touched the side of her face. "Where's your mom today? No, wait, don't tell me." He looked at Jimmy. "Jewel's place?"

Jimmy nodded.

"Jeez-Louise." He looked back at Leah. "You two still squattin' in that warehouse down on Eleventh?"

"Uh-huh. It's not too bad there."

"She's got no business keeping you in a place like that and usin' her money to buy—"

"Merc," said Jimmy, a warning.

"I can't help it," shouted Merc, rising to his feet. "Shit, when I was workin' over in Panama a couple years ago, we'd been hired to blow a worthless fuck like Jewel right out of his socks. Him, and about forty of his boys. I enjoyed it a little too much, y' know? Won't do for a merc to start takin' sides. That's how come I got out."

"I know," said Jimmy.

Merc smiled, and it wasn't a nice smile. "Still got me a little firepower." He looked around, nervous, then pulled open one side of his jacket to reveal a large silver 9mm semiautomatic tucked into the waist of his pants.

"Oh, great," said Jimmy, "look at this: *Son of the Equalizer*—close your coat, for chrissakes. People will think you're flashing us."

"Hey, if I decided to whip out the man-meat," said Merc, closing his coat, "you'd *know* you been flashed. Didn't mean to shock you, Leah."

"You didn't."

Jimmy laughed.

Merc pulled himself up straight. "Gettin' off the point here a bit, ain't we? I'd just *love* to dust our little Jewel. 'Bout the only way we'd ever get Denise away from him. And you know, don't you, Chief, that it's gotta be us. Nobody else give's a rat's ass. We're just partial people to all of them, and you don't pay no attention to a partial person."

"My father had a term for us," said Jimmy. "He called people like us Hollow Houses, the Unbelonging: vessels with homeless spirits."

"We don't belong here," said Merc.

"We should be somewhere else," whispered Jimmy.

And Leah thought: *someone come.*

"Well, Darlin'," said Merc, laying a hand on top of Leah's head, "I imagine your mom's gonna be havin' herself a private little party tonight. Maybe Jimmy and me—bet'cha didn't think I knew your real name, did'ya, Jimmy?—maybe the two of us'll cruise on by in the Chiefmobile later and see how you're doing. Can't never tell how a person's gonna act after they shoot that shit into their veins." He saw something behind them, then rolled his eyes. "Speaking of shit . . ."

"Watch it, Merc," said Jimmy. "I'm serious."

"Leah!" shouted Mommy, trying to sound nice and almost making it. "C'mon, hon. Time to get something to eat."

"Bitch's gonna buy her daughter some real *food?*" whispered Merc to Jimmy. "Sorry state, when junkies start thinking of others. Almost enough to make you believe there's a God."

"Put a sock in it, will you?" said Jimmy.

Mommy came up behind Leah and grabbed her arm. "Say good-bye to your friends, hon. You can maybe come back tomorrow."

"How's Jewel doing?" said Merc.

"Fine," snapped Mommy. "He said to send his regards."

"I'll bet," muttered Jimmy.

"You see Denise?" asked Leah.

"Oh, she, uh . . . she wasn't feeling too well today, hon. Jewel was making her stay in bed."

Jimmy snorted a nasty laugh. "What a lovely way to put it."

Mommy pushed Leah behind her. "All right, assholes, you've had your fun. I don't need this shit from the likes of you. Nice crate, by the way."

"That's the Chiefmobile, Mommy!"

"It's a goddamned orange crate, for hauling garbage." And she turned around and pulled Leah along.

Leah managed to turn around and wave at Jimmy and Merc. They waved back, but didn't look very happy.

As they got to the corner, Leah looked over at Jewel's building and saw Denise standing at her window. She looked pale and empty and sad. The lower half of the window was foggy with steam, and Denise was drawing patterns in the condensation with her finger. When she finished her drawing, she knelt down and looked out through the two opposing almond-shapes.

Below the almonds, she'd written: *someone come.*

Leah wanted to touch her, to tell Denise that she'd be her friend.

Buddy would like Denise; Merc and Jimmy, too.

Partial people; Hollow Houses.

"Who will take me?" Leah whispered.

"What?" snapped Mommy.

"Nothin'."

"Christ Almighty. Fuckin' *starchild.* Airhead's more like it."

"I'm sorry, Mommy."

"Not half as much as I am. C'mon. I suppose we should get you something to eat. Just eat it quick. I need to get back."

"Yes, Mommy."

V

Leah finished untying the funny rubber band from around her mother's arm and threw it on top of the box they kept all their clothes in. Leah didn't understand why her mother always left that thing around her arm; she had lots of time to take it all the way off after the needle-thing but she never did: she just loosened it enough so the vein would go back down after she stuck the needle in. Then she shook a lot and made weird noises, sighing and growling at the same time. A lot of the time Leah even had to take the needle out of her mother's arm after Mommy went to sleep sort-of and that made her nervous because she was afraid she might slip and Mommy would start to bleed too much and maybe die. She didn't like these nights because Mommy wasn't her mother anymore, she was like some zombie from those old black-and-white horror movies Jewel watched on his television. Mommy knew a lot of zombies; they always came around to see her after the dark-coat man gave her money for her babies.

They all had black eyes and runny noses and were shaky and smelled like old hamburger. Their skin was gray and crusty and all of them had the same little hole-bruises on their arms. They would give Mommy a little money or food or something for a "taste" of the needle-stuff and then light the candles. Leah thought that part was kind of pretty; all of them sitting huddled over the candles, heating up the shiny spoons and lighting the sticks that smelled like Christmas trees. They would laugh and tell jokes and the candle flames made them all look like broken dolls, and it was kind of soft and glowing . . . but then they'd take out the needles and those funny rubber bands that they wrapped around their arms and it wasn't pretty anymore.

That's when Leah would leave to go see Buddy.

Just like tonight. She was glad that Mommy had done the needle-thing by herself because that meant Leah didn't have to worry about someone else trying to stop her, so she wadded up some old clothes and put them under her mother's head for a pillow, covered her with an old rug so she wouldn't get too cold, and silently crept to the bottom of the stairs. This was fun, like she was in one of those old movies where they were escaping from jail. She reached the bottom of the stairs and walked straight ahead into the middle of the basement where a bunch of barrels were stacked up, then pushed one of them aside and crawled through the opening, careful not to jostle anything and make the stack come crashing down. In the middle of the floor was a loose board, and Leah slid it to one side. This part was never hard to do, the warehouse was all stinking and falling apart, anyway, like all the buildings around here. There were probably all kinds of loose boards that she could rip up, but she didn't want to. This was her special board, her special secret; she had first seen Buddy's lights glowing from underneath this loose board, and because she wanted to keep it a secret, she had stacked all the barrels around it like a bunch of pop cans so no one else would be able to find it. She didn't ever want Mommy to find out about Buddy because then she'd probably tell the dark-coat man about it and Leah just *knew* that dark-coat man had been talking about Buddy when asked about her having *any other friends.*

Sometimes she felt like she had to be scared all the time.

She couldn't stop thinking about what Mommy had said to her, about letting Jewel take her up to his room. That hurt Leah because she loved her mother very, very much.

She squeezed through the opening left by the missing board, and once she was inside, turned around and pulled the board back into place. This way, no one would ever be able to find her. The way she felt right now, Leah wasn't sure she ever wanted to go back to her mother; maybe if she didn't come back, Mommy would know how she felt when she was left alone all the time.

In the darkness Leah could hear the sounds of rats running back and forth. That was good, because it meant the rats were scared and *that* meant that Buddy was waiting for her.

She scooted over onto her butt and slid down the dirt incline. This part was fun, too; it was like going down the slide at one of the playgrounds Mommy let her play on once. Even though she'd only been able to go down the slide one time, Leah never forgot what it felt like because it made her think that she was going home; the speed, the feeling that she could take flight at any moment, the wind pressing against her—wherever she was supposed to be instead of here, she'd found some small part of it that day on the sliding board.

She hit the bottom of the sub-basement with a moist thud and heard the rats screech and run into the deeper darkness. It was hard to see down here, so she got on her hands and knees and moved forward very slowly. This was the hard part, making sure she didn't get all mixed-up in the dark. She slid her hands forward, then dragged her legs; once, twice, three times, and on the third time she felt the cold metal under her fingers.

The door to the Rusty Room.

She took a deep breath and rose up on her knees—she had to be strong for this because the door was heavy—and worked her fingers into a crack right along the top and pulled.

The door came up with a loud *screech* sound that felt like an icepick stuck in her ears. She fell back, panting, then held her breath and listened; she always expected Mommy to wake up when the door made that noise and come looking for her.

But she never did. It was like all she cared about was her needle-thing and not about where Leah was.

She crawled forward once again and peered down; there was a little light tonight, sort of red-blue, and that was enough for her to see the rounded walls of the metal tunnel, so she scooted around, slid her legs in, and pushed forward, sliding down the metal tunnel and laughing. She couldn't help laughing; this was fun, even more fun than the sliding board.

She landed on the floor and slid forward a few more feet because the floor of the Rusty Room was made out of black glass; at least, that's what it looked like to Leah. In the middle of the room was a tall pillar that narrowed in the center and supported part of the domed ceiling. The walls were made out of some kind of metal that was very old and had started rusting over the years; the room smelled like dust and copper, and sometimes when Leah would touch one of the walls, the rust came off on her hands, revealing layers upon layers of much older rust underneath. In one of the corners of the room—and it puzzled Leah that a room so round would actually have squared corners—was a hole that looked like something had exploded there. One time she stuck her head through the hole and saw the River of Ash-People that went on and on, farther than she could see even with a flashlight. Buddy had told her that the Ash-People weren't all people, some of them were animals and other creatures that *didn't quite work out as planned.* She wasn't sure she knew what Buddy meant by that, but, still, they were all pretty neat, like sand sculptures people made at the beach in summer. From what she understood, the Ash-People had all gotten caught in some kind of fire-flood, like volcano lava, and had been washed down here where they were forever frozen in one position when the lava hardened.

It seemed kind of sad to her that all of the Ash-People looked like they were reaching upward, hoping someone would pull them out and take them home because they didn't really belong *here.* She wondered if that mammoth Merc talked about had been reaching up when the scientists found it.

She decided not to say hello to the Ash-People tonight, and hoped they'd understand. She had important things to talk about with Buddy.

Then she noticed that Buddy had written some more words on the wall above the hole:

someone come
be there in the morning
when I
wake up
with your silver thread
to lead me out
I don't belong here
who will take me?

someone come

A few feet away from the central pillar was a doorway, and above the door there was a sign of somc sort, printed in raised letters (she *guessed* they were letters, anyway; she'd never seen anything quite like them), that shone with an almost eerie phosphorescence, just like all those neon signs downtown where Jewel lived. The red-blue light she'd seen from above earlier came from those letters, and gave off enough light that she could make her way around the Rusty Room without banging into anything—not that there was much to bang into; just a large white table like in a doctor's office, and a bunch of things that looked like leather coffins stacked one on top of the other.

"Buddy?" she called softly.

And waited to be answered by music that was both primitive and majestic; clicks, grunts, wheezing whistles, then a series of trills, arpeggios, and multi-toned flutings: all parts of Buddy's language. A long time ago, when she'd first met him, Buddy had put her on the table and done something to her head with a gizmo that looked like one of those things doctors looked in your ears with, only Buddy's gizmo had a kind of liquidy spring attached that uncoiled like a snake and went into her ears and then deeper. It had tickled a lot, but ever since then Leah had been able to understand what Buddy was saying to her.

"I know I'm late. I'm sorry, but Mommy . . . Mommy sold the baby tonight and then we had to go and get some of her needle-stuff."

Still, she was answered by silence. That was all

right, though; sometimes Buddy didn't feel like talking *or* showing himself. It was enough for Leah to just know he was around. She could feel him near.

"I got a bag of King Dons the doctor gave me!" She pulled the crushed bag from under her shirt. "Uh-oh. They got squished. But that's okay, they still taste real good, they're just kinda messy." She worked the remains of one from its package and held it out. "You want one? I saved a package for you."

Silence.

"Okay, if you're sure. I'll probably eat 'em all. I'm still kinda hungry. Mommy bought me a hamburger but I didn't get to eat it all 'cause she was in a hurry." She shrugged. "It was kinda greasy, anyway."

She devoured the first package of cakes, then opened the next one. "I wish you weren't so quiet tonight, Buddy. I missed you. Mommy, she . . . I dunno. I think she does that needle-thing because she's sad about something and it won't leave her alone. Sometimes, when she talks about how she first met my daddy, she gets all sad, then mean. I don't really understand a lot about it. I don't get what a metal cave is supposed to be, unless it's something like your place. Buddy. I guess maybe that's it, and maybe that's what makes her sad enough to do the needle-thing. I bet that's why all of them do the needle-thing, to make the sad go away. I just wish . . ." She wiped her eyes, surprised that she'd started crying again.

"I just wish that she didn't have to give the babies to the dark-coat man for money. She gave him my little sister. I never had a little sister before and I didn't even get to name her.

"I wish you'd say something. You're my best-best friend. I love you, Buddy."

She was answered only by silence, but in that silence she felt Buddy's confusion; not at her being sad, or hungry, or about Mommy and the babies and the needle-stuff, but at one word: love. It wasn't that Buddy didn't know what love was, because he did, in his way; what confused him was that Leah felt such deep and strong affection for him.

"Okay, I g-guess you don't feel like company tonight. I'll come back again tomorrow night, okay? I'll save you some of the King Dons, in case you change your mind." She made her way over to the metal tunnel and saw that Buddy had, as usual, turned it into a ladder so she could climb back up.

She started up, then swung out, one hand still gripping a rung, and waved good-night to the Ash-People.

Above the hole, some new words had been written:

and where do I live?
in the empty spaces where
a spirit should be
among the odd, damaged ones
in hollow houses of flesh
and bone
that the Belonging will not
see

someone come
one last time
I will wait for you
you ask who will take me?

someone come
and answer

soon

tomorrow

within the cell, life is long, life is hard.
within the cell, life is hard.

and home is a cruel joke.

someone come.

"Okay," said Leah, smiling. "I'll come back tomorrow."

VI

Mommy was awake when Leah got back, but there was a man with her and they were doing the grabbing thing. Leah hated that because Mommy always screamed a lot when she did the grabbing thing with a man, but she knew that the grabbing thing was how babies were made because Long Red had told her about it once, because that's what hookers did, except they didn't want to have babies so they just did it for fun. Like Mommy sometimes did with one of her needle-friends.

Leah sat in a dark corner where they couldn't see her, listening to her mother moan and scream and say fuck-me-yes-yes.

Leah cried, wishing that Buddy had felt like company.

VII

After it was over, Leah watched as her mother and the man lay naked in the candlelight, sweating. She hoped that the grabbing thing was over because she was getting hungry again. Maybe Mommy would be in a good mood now and give her some money so she could buy a hot dog or taco or something.

She walked out of the darkness and the man laying next to her mother sat up and smiled.

"So that's her, huh, babe?"

"Yeah . . ."

"Wow. I ain't never seen a . . . a whatchamacall-it—space-baby before."

"Not much to look at, is she?"

"Hey, I think she's real pretty. Like her mom."

"Mommy's just a former abductee."

"Yeah, but them saucer-men must've got them-selves a real taste for that nice Earth-snatch of yours, what with them always asking those dudes to bring you back so they can have some more."

"Fuck you."

"You just did."

"Oh, yeah, now I remember." They laughed, and Leah laughed, too, then came over and stood next to Mommy and said, "Can I have some money to buy a hot dog?"

"You already ate once today."

"Please?"

Mommy jumped up and slapped her hard across the mouth, knocking Leah back into the boxes.

"I said no!"

" 'Kay," whimpered Leah, wiping the blood from her chin and trying hard not to cry.

"Her blood's the same color as ours," said the man.

"So what?"

"So, I dunno . . . it's interesting, that's all."

"Shit! Only reason I keep her is because they give me more money each time to make sure I don't accidentally leave her someplace. But that ends next month. She'll be six then, and I guess there's something that happens to them when they turn six, something important, so they're gonna take her to the Center."

"But you said they was gonna take you, too."

"Do I look stupid? I know damn well that when they show up to get us, there're gonna be *two* cars 'cause they'll want us to ride separate, and *hers'll* be the only car with a passenger when they get there. I mean, it ain't like they couldn't still use me, but Mr. I'm-In-Charge, he don't like me so much."

The man *hmmm*'d, then picked up one of the needles. "And this shit don't have no effect on the babies?"

"Nope. They've all been real healthy."

The man looked at Leah. "You ever do any experimentin' on her?"

"Like what?"

"Ever send her tripping?"

Leah wondered then, for the first time, if the needle-thing was their way of Removing themselves from what was going on around them.

Mommy looked at her and smiled. "It's not like *I have* to take care of her now, is it? They won't be giving me any more money."

"I hear Mexico's real pretty this time of year. You 'n' me, we take your money and your stash, we maybe hit Jewel's for some extra, then head on down. We could set ourselves up pretty good."

Mommy threw off the rug she'd been using for a blanket. "She's been nothing but a pain in the ass since she was born. Let's do it."

Mommy's eyes looked just like the dark-coat man's and Leah tried to get to her feet and run away but she was still dizzy from being hit so hard and Mommy and the man were on top of her before she could even stand up straight and one of them hit her real hard in the mouth with a fist and everything went white and then she felt the rubber band being tied around her arm and then a sting and she cried out for Buddy to come and save her but then the world went liquid and runny and numb . . .

VIII

She was back at the Wall of Skulls, only now the skulls had grown flesh and become faces again, and all of them were talking but no sound emerged from their mouths; all she could hear were tings and buzzes and beeps. Climbing on the faces, she made her way up to the top of the wall where a woolly mammoth stood in front of a pinball machine, concentrating for all it was worth. She said hello and it looked over its shoulder at her. It had Buddy's black-almond eyes. "Come on," it said. "I'm getting tired. You take over for me."

Leah stood in front of the pinball machine and placed her hands on the buttons. Even though she wasn't doing anything, the machine went crazy; lights blinking, silver balls shooting all over the place and bouncing off the bumpers, the score ding-ding-dinging higher and higher, and she began to remove her hands but the mammoth said, "No, just keep a grip on the machine and it'll continue to work." So she did.

The mammoth stood next to her and pointed with its trunks to a field that lay beyond the wall. "Everything dies," it said, "but we only know about it as a kind of abstraction. If you were to go out into that field and stand in the middle, almost everything you can see is in the process of dying, and most of those things will be dead long before you are. If it weren't for the constant renewal and replacement going on before your eyes—even though you can't see most of it—the whole world would turn to stone and sand underneath your feet. Everything dies. But there are some things that do not seem to die at all; they simply vanish totally into their own progeny." The mammoth paused for a moment to munch on a few buttercups.

"Single cells do this," it said. "Not eat buttercups, but vanish into their progeny. The cell becomes two, then four, and so on, until after a while the last trace is gone. But you can't look upon that as death; barring unnatural mutations that should be gotten rid of, the descendants are simply that first cell, living over and over again. And sometimes, if things go as planned, eventu-

ally the descendants will grow back into *their original form; they will* re-*become the first cell.*

"Do you understand what's happening right now?"

"No," said Leah, watching as the stars above came closer, grew colder.

"Buddy is what you were before you became what you are, and he is also what you will become again one day, if things go as planned."

"Why didn't I just stay like Buddy?"

It was so cold, suddenly; so very, very cold.

"If I knew the answer to that, none of this would have ever happened. But I think it has something to do with worthiness."

The mammoth screamed as the ice came . . .

IX

"The bitch! I'll kill her, I swear to God!" Merc, screaming.

"Not if I get my hands on her first, you won't." Jimmy, crying.

Leah tried to move, tried to say something, but her body was stiff and cold and rigid; she couldn't even blink her eyes.

Am I dead? She wondered, then figured she must be or else Merc and Jimmy wouldn't be acting this way.

Merc pulled out the 9mm. "I'll bet you anything that cunt went over to Jewel's to get herself a little more candy before she takes off."

Some things do not seem to die at all.

"Jesus—Merc! Get back here!"

"What is it?"

"She's . . . God almighty, *she's still alive!* Here, feel her pulse—no, in her neck!"

"Oh god . . ."

"Christ, Merc, I don't know what to do."

"Thought you were a medicine man?"

"Sachem! I was a *sachem* in training! A *spiritual* healer."

"Oh."

Jimmy lifted Leah's body into his arms. "C'mon, Merc, pull me out of here. We gotta find a cab and get her to the hospi—"

"Oh God!"

"What? Merc, you're scaring me, what're you looking—"

"Over there! In the light! Oh God!"

A breeze, old and tired.

A touch, warm and safe.

Fingers, long and willowy.

Light.

So much almond-eyes light . . .

X

The stars began to fade like guttering candles, snuffed out one by one. Out in the depths of space the great celestial cities, the galaxies, cluttered with the memorabilia of ages, were dying. Tens of billions of years passed in the growing darkness. Occasional flickers of light pierced the fall of cosmic night, and only spurts of activity delayed the sentence of a universe condemned from the beginning to become a galactic graveyard. Light flowed inward, and the sky snowed a blizzard of galaxies as the lens of night burned brighter than the sun, than all the stars in supernova, and the human race fell on its knees, blinded forever by the white-hot darkness in its eyes.

The air crackled with rage.

"I will do this for you, if you want me to," said a voice. "They deserve nothing better, yet they deserve so much more."

"Buddy?"

"Shhh. Just tell me what to do."

"Be here in the morning when I wake up."

"If that's what you want."

"Can't you ever go back?"

"This is home. It always has been."

"I'm sorry."

"I know. Thank you."

"For what?"

"For teaching me about worthiness. And love."

"Am I dead, Buddy?"

"No. But the time is upon us to fly."

Leah smiled. "Like Jimmy's song."

"Yes, like Jimmy's song."

And then Leah felt herself freed from her body, everywhere and nowhere at the same time, becoming light in its truest meaning, becoming light in its purest intention, including the darkness, and for a moment she was aware of a coldness that transcended temperature, a chilling sense of timelessness that touched her mind rather than her flesh, and within that coldness she heard an echo—distant but strong—of utter loneliness, and she recognized this sound because she'd been hearing it in the back of her own mind for all her life, only now it was fading away, away, away as the empty space left in its wake was filled with a blossoming awareness of all the knowledge left behind by the descendants who had simply been the first cell living over and over again, and though she didn't yet understand everything revealed to her, she smiled deep within herself, knowing she would *understand, in time . . .*

XI

She awoke on the table in the Rusty Room and rolled over to see Jimmy and Merc standing beside her.

"How're you feeling?" said Jimmy, reaching out to touch her, then pulling his hand back at the last moment.

"I feel okay," said Leah. "You don't gotta worry about touching me."

"I know," said Jimmy, "it's just that . . . well, the last time I touched you—" He took a step backward, and only then did Leah realize that Jimmy was . . . standing.

"Oh, Jimmy—"

"You did this," he said. "You gave my legs back to me."

She rose up on the table and looked at Merc. "Can I do anything for you, Merc?"

"You two're gonna have to . . . to give me a little while to get my mind around all of this." He leaned over and brushed some of Leah's hair out of her eyes. "You sure you're feeling all right?"

"Uh-huh. Did you guys meet Buddy?"

Merc looked at Jimmy. "Well, I guess you could say that. Dude made himself quite an entrance."

Leah giggled. "I'll bet you were scared, huh?"

"No," said Merc. "I *been* scared. This was *way* past that."

"I damn near fainted," said Jimmy, then, looking around, added: "Where is he now?"

Leah smiled. "He went home. Sort-of." She jumped down from the table and walked over and gave Jimmy a hug. It felt *great* to hug him standing up!

Jimmy kissed the top of her head, then stroked her hair. "What do you want to do now?"

"I want to go get Denise."

Merc smiled. "Do we have to be nice about it to Jewel?"

Leah's smile grew wider. "No. Jewel isn't Worthy."

Jimmy and Merc looked at each other.

"Then we're gonna find Long Red," said Leah. "And all the others just like us. And the dark-coat man. I want my brothers and my little sister back."

"You sure you're up to this?" said Jimmy.

"Uh-huh. I will take care of you. I will help us all make a home."

Jimmy tilted her head back with his hands and looked into her eyes. *"Peye'wik?"*

"No," said Leah. "It Is *Here*."

"Well, what're we waiting for?" said Merc, pulling out the 9mm and jacking back the slide. "Let's get this invasion started."

They made their way over to the ladder. Jimmy went first, then Merc, and Leah went last.

But before she began to climb, she crossed over to the hole to say good-bye to the River of Ash-People, then read the last words Buddy had left for her on the wall:

someone come
give this body no limits
slough the fevers
with your cool hand

make the flesh home

within the skin, life is long, life is hard
within the skin, life is hard

but not for much longer.

where do I live?
someone come

who will take me?

Leah looked down at the black-glass floor and saw her reflection; for just an instant, long enough for her to know for sure, she saw her face become two, one superimposed on top of the other, and smiled as she looked into the black-almond eyes that watched the world from behind her own.

She pressed her finger into the rust and wrote:

I am here
someone's come
I will take you.

"No more living in Hollow Houses," she whispered. "We'll make ourselves Worthy again. I promise."

She thought she heard the Ash-People singing thanks.

Then left to join her waiting friends.

The invasion was about to begin.

And a little child would lead them.

RADIANCE

Nina Kiriki Hoffman

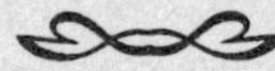

YOU KNOW HOW YOU OBJECT TO LAWS IN PRINCIPLE, distantly and without heat, until they come home to you?

I would have voted against any law that gave the Radiants rights to our corpses, but we didn't get to vote on it; Congress passed it, and that was that. It became a box you could check on the back of your driver's license. Medical donor. Alien donor. It was up to each individual.

They could have done it differently, those politicians. They could have. But they didn't.

Energy politics. Cheap power. Pollutionless fuel. A lot of the big PACs fought it, but when we saw how other countries who signed on with the Radiants earlier than we did were about to outstrip us in technology and production, I guess maybe we had to go with the new law.

I don't want the aliens playing with my body after I'm gone. Cremation, that's the death-style for Judy D'Angelo.

My sister Carla felt differently.

Once the Radiants get our bodies, they're supposed to move them to someplace on the other side of the world, where there's less chance of encountering people who knew the bodies in life. So there was no reason for me to ever run into Carla after she died. I'm not a traveler. I've spent all my life within fifty miles of where I was born.

Most of the Radiants we have in Sparrow Creek look like they come from East India, rules about relocation being what they are. They have their own enclave on the far side of the creek away from the rest of town. They do some mixing, though not a whole lot. You see them in the Quick Lunch Diner and at the library and hanging around the bus station. Sometimes they're at the public pool in the summer—guess they get hot same as we do—but when they get into the pool, most regular people get out.

I don't know. There's just something creepy about swimming with corpses.

Skin goes gray after death; that's one of the systems the Radiants don't repair just right, though from rumors, I hear they get everything else in the bodies working as well as or better than it did in life. My husband, Tony, has a theory about Radiant skin color. He has a lot of theories, and he likes to tell me about them.

You can always tell a Radiant from that gray skin, and also from the light in the eyes, as though the

Radiants just can't stop themselves from shining, even though they clothe themselves in flesh.

I saw some Radiants without bodies when I was a little girl.

I had hiked down the creek a ways toward where the water got pinched into a rock canyon and ran faster. There was a big flat rock out that way I used to do some dreaming on. I had to wade to it, surrounded as it was by moving water on all sides.

I was there at twilight, having left a Fourth of July picnic before we even got to the fireworks. Carla had been teasing me again about being stupid. It was true she got all the good grades, and it was true that when she teased me I just turned red and couldn't get my mouth to say anything smart back, so I felt stupider and stupider, as though she put a spell on me with every taunt.

I ran away, and waded to my dreaming rock on the underwater rocks I knew as well as anything my bare feet had ever touched, and I sat there as night crept out of all the places it hides during the day. The rock was still warm from leftover sun, and the air was summer-dusty and water-wet.

So I kept looking toward the fairgrounds, where the rest of my family was probably still scarfing homemade ice cream and chocolate chip cookies, maybe even roasting marshmallows, and where the fireworks would bloom eventually. They wouldn't miss me. I was too stupid to bother with.

The floating lights came to me there on my dreaming rock.

I didn't hear them. I noticed flickering near my feet

and turned to look over my shoulder down the canyon and there they were, drifting a few feet above the stream, flickers of light reflecting off the water below them.

One was purple as a spring violet, a cluster of dark purple lights with lighter purple streamers up and down; one was yellow as firelight, a big smudge of light like a giant reverse fingerprint hanging in the air; and one was pale pale blue as the edge of sky just after dawn, spiky with light as a porcupine is with quills.

Radiants had only been on Earth about three years then, during what people called the First Phase, in hindsight—they could come and go at will as long as they didn't hurt anybody. Not that we knew how to stop them from doing whatever they wanted. How do you cage an energy creature? How do you hurt one? That was before the Radiants made the deal for bodies with various world governments; at that point, none of us knew what they really wanted. Linguists could communicate with them, but the rest of us couldn't.

All I knew in that moment was that they were beautiful.

I swiped away the tears that blurred my vision and stared at the lights, not quite sure what they were. I had seen a few stories in the paper—Carla liked talking about the Radiants for current events—but I had never seen Radiants before. Fireworks that didn't burn themselves out?

They drifted closer. Over the chuckle of the creek I could hear a faint humming sound, not a human hum but more like wind going through wires.

They stared at me and I stared at them for a long time. Parts of them shifted and spun, but they stayed pretty much in the same space they had started in; no drift of disintegration.

At last the purple one stretched out a ray of light and touched my face with it. I was so lost in dreaming wonder that at first I didn't think anything about it. The light touched my cheek like my mother's fingertip, soft and warm.

The warmth seeped into my face and spread under the skin. I still dreamed, but now I dreamed that something asked me questions, and I gave answers. I thought about Carla, about Mom and Dad, about our cousins; about the cool bite of pink lemonade in the mouth on a hot afternoon, and about roasting hot dogs over a coal fire, how they sizzled, and how the first bite was too hot but wonderful, juicy and charred; about what Carla had said to me before I ran away from the picnic, and how I had felt hearing it, the fire that had burned in my face, the way my throat had closed on tears.

I liked remembering the tastes, and the good way the sun warmed me on hot summer days, but thinking about Carla calling me stupid made me cry all over again, and I didn't like that.

I woke from my dream and clapped my hand over my cheek.

The purple light stopped shining directly at me.

I was afraid of them then. I knelt on the edge of my rock and splashed water on my face, trying to wash away the alien heat. I was afraid to look up. What if they shone into my eyes and blinded me? What if they wanted more from me, the secret dreams of rage I had after I turned the lights out at night, the sick miserable feeling in the pit of my stomach after I had told a lie to Mom about who had really eaten the chocolate cake? I didn't want any more questions that I would answer before I decided whether I wanted to answer.

I lay face down on the rock, shielding my face with my hands, for a long time. When at last I looked up, the lights had disappeared.

My husband, Tony, is a psychologist. He says the Radiants keep their skin gray because they want us to know what they are. He says if they blended better they would scare us more. As long as we can identify them we don't have to be afraid that they're sneaking around doing things we can't understand.

So I was more than startled when I saw Carla again six months after her funeral. Her skin was the wrong color.

I was in the Quick Lunch having my usual pastrami on rye and watching the other secretary from the insurance office where I work, Arlene, eat a salad. She hates salads, but she always eats them. She was talking about her cat, Puffball, who does more cute things than you would think a cat could.

"He's learning to open doors," she said.

"Imagine," I said. Which was mostly what I said when talking to Arlene. I lifted my coffee mug off the circle of light on the table that kept it just the right temperature, and took a sip.

"Reaches up and turns the knob. It works better if

he's on the side of the door he can push when he gets it open. But he can tug on the bottom of the door if he has to."

"Imagine."

"I have to tell you, it's starting to spook me," she said. "I don't want the cat to be able to open doors. I want him to stay where I put him."

I glanced over and saw that in the next booth there was a woman all in black, wearing a black broad-brimmed straw hat with a heavy black veil. But behind the veil, where her eyes should be, there were two spots of purple glow, staring at me.

I looked at her hands and they were pink. Pink fingers clutched a mug of coffee tight. Coffee steam rose past her veiled face.

How could she drink through that veil?

Radiants don't like the taste of coffee, only the smell.

Alien and not gray. Something wrong with that picture.

"What do you think I should do?" Arlene said.

"Huh?" I turned back to her, watched her eat the last bite of salad.

"The cat can open *doors*, Judy. Aren't you listening?"

"Lock them," I said, remembering a purple touch on my face and mental doors I had not been able to close. In the twenty-five years since I had met the Radiants at the creek, I had avoided them, both during Phase One, exploration, and Phase Two, corpse occupation. I never met their eyes. I didn't want to look at the light. I didn't want them seeing who I was inside.

Nobody in any of the news stories during Phase One had talked about experiences similar to what had happened to me. No lights reaching out to touch a person's face, no mind-opening. I sometimes thought I had made it up.

"I don't want to live like that," Arlene said. "I want to go from one room to the next without having to unlock doors. Maybe if I just lock the front door all the time . . ."

The woman in black touched my shoulder. "Judy," she said in a low voice.

I startled like a fly-bitten horse.

"Excuse me," said the veiled woman. "I didn't mean to frighten you." She didn't take her hand off my shoulder, though.

"Someone you know?" Arlene asked.

"No," I said. My voice came out strained. Shock seeped through me. I was staring at the hand on my shoulder, at the long pudgy fingers, the half-moon nails. Carla's capable hand, last seen in the temporary coffin the Sparrow Creek Mortuary used as though it were a hotel room: put the corpses in for viewing, take them out and hand them over to the Radiants, fluff the satin for the next corpse.

Or perhaps the Radiants were already at work inside the corpses while they were being viewed. I wasn't sure what the procedure was.

"We need to get back to work," Arlene said, lowering her salad plate into the green pool of light in the center of the table. We had both already thumbed the small pink light patches at our places that registered our thumb prints and extracted money from our access accounts to pay for our meals.

Smart light. What the Radiants had traded us for our dead.

"I have to talk to you," said the woman.

I kept my eyes down. "I can't imagine being interested in anything you have to say," I said. I astonished myself. I never would have had the courage to talk that way to Carla while she was alive.

"She doesn't have time to talk to you," Arlene said. I felt an upwelling of gratitude toward her. The hand on my shoulder seemed to have paralyzed me. "We have to go back to work."

"I'll pay for your time," said the woman.

"Please," said Arlene, "what do you take us for? Come on, Judy!" She reached past the woman in black, grasped my hand, pulled me to my feet. The woman's hand slid from my shoulder.

Arlene and I ran out of the restaurant.

Our office was only two doors away, but we were both panting by the time we got there. "Thanks," I said to her. "Thanks, Arlene."

"Who was that? Did you know her?"

"Did you see her eyes?" I asked.

"How could I see anything through that veil?"

I hesitated. A Radiant who wasn't gray? This might be the start of a huge scandal. Or maybe not. Maybe there was no law that said the Radiants had to be gray. Maybe they just did it to keep us pacified, like Tony said.

A Radiant who used to be Carla.

My aggravating sister.

My sister.

A Radiant. No one I knew.

But still . . . Carla.

"I can't explain yet," I said.

Arlene frowned at me, then shrugged and said, "All right."

The Radiant was waiting for me when I got off at four-thirty. Arlene took a different light-bus home, so she wasn't there to save me this time.

"Judy," said the Radiant.

"What do you want?" I asked.

"Just to talk to you."

"My husband will be waiting for me." Actually Tony's last appointment on Thursdays ended at six, and we didn't have that much to say to each other anyway, unless he had come up with a new theory of something.

"Please," it said.

It might be the sort to wait around until I said yes. Wait across the street and watch the house while I was home. Wait at my bus stop in the morning. Wait in the restaurant while I ate lunch. Wait here, on the street near the office, when I got off.

Might as well get this over with.

It was summer in Sparrow Creek, and though the Radiants had taught us how to augment the atmosphere and tame weather into useful storms and modified sun, it was still hot in the late afternoon. I headed down the sidewalk toward the fairgrounds, thinking of the picnic tables there, neutral ground, where no one I knew was likely to see me talking to this—thing.

"Aren't you supposed to be on the other side of the world?" I asked it as it walked beside me.

"In one reality," it said.

"What, now we have more than one reality?"

"It is time for another shift."

"Phase Three? What's Phase Three going to be? Who decides stuff like that?"

"It is part of a repeating pattern of contact," it said.

"Why tell me? I'm less than nothing to you. I'm not even a donor. I don't want you . . . things inside me."

"Just making conversation," it said, which seemed very strange to me.

It followed me across the summer-browned grass to the picnic table where I had eaten twenty-five summers before, the table I had run away from because of Carla. I brushed off the bench and sat down. Nothing here had been modernized. You couldn't touch a pool of light and order food or water. Here was just stained and somewhat splintery wood with initials and cuss words carved into it.

The Radiant sat across from me and lifted off its hat and veil.

And it was Carla. Her chipmunk cheeks, sagging a little with middle age, her freckled pug nose, her expressive mouth with the full lower lip; her broad, thinker's forehead and her heavy, wavy chestnut hair, just another thing I had envied her, because my hair was too fine and never grew long, and it was a lighter color of brown called dishwater.

Her eyes had changed. A lavender swirl of light had replaced the iris in each eye.

"So talk," I said.

"Do you recognize me?" it asked.

"What are you talking about? I don't know you from . . . from starlight."

"We met not far from here." It turned and glanced at the creek through the trees, and then south, toward the canyon where my dreaming rock had been.

"What?" I touched my cheek, remembering the three wild Radiants I had seen. I had told no one about them.

"What I did to you, that was against the rules of early contact."

I squinted at the face that used to be my sister's. It didn't have any real expression, and the voice, too, was flat. I had overheard Radiants talking to people—in the market, in restaurants. They could mimic human speech perfectly if they wanted to. They could use facial muscles to communicate the emotions we expected from them, as though they had the same palette of feelings we had. I had never been sure how real it was for them, but then, I hadn't wanted to get close enough to test it. I had let Tony tell me what he thought about them. It wasn't the same as knowing.

I shrugged. "So what?" I said.

"So who are you now?" It sounded curious and worried.

It was strange to look into my sister's face and see someone else. The restless, crushing intelligence was gone, the impatience with anyone around her slower than she, the casual cruelty and constant questions. She had always been too swift to slow down for answers, as though she'd lose momentum and was afraid she would never regain it. She had died in Tasmania, researching something forest related, and her body had been brought home just long enough for us to have a memorial, and then back she went, newly inhabited, to the other side of the world.

I thought.

I said, "If you're the one who touched me, how did you end up inside my sister? That seems beyond coincidence."

It nodded. "It was planned. I broke a rule. I must make reparations."

"Really?"

It nodded again.

"What does that mean? Reparations to who? Me?"

"Yes."

I wondered if it would let me set my sister on fire and dance around her while she burned. But that seemed like too much trouble, and not very likely. "What kind of reparations?"

It clasped its hands, placed them on the tabletop. Its forehead furrowed. "Who are you now?" it asked.

"What business is it of yours?"

"I need to know how I hurt you so I can do whatever is possible to made amends."

I shook my head. "What you did to me didn't change me," I said. "I'm just who I am. A wife. A secretary. A daughter, a sister. A friend."

"Do you feel stupid?" it asked, and it was Carla's voice to the life, the undertone of sneer.

I looked at her. Her eyes were brown again. There was no sign of Radiant in her. My throat swelled and closed. I wondered what I had done to bring such torture down on me, to have her gone, and now to have her back. I felt the heat of tears in my eyes, the heat of flush on my face.

When she went away to college I began to have a life of my own, but every time she came back she sliced through any threads of progress or independence I had woven in her absence, and she came back just often enough to keep me from building any strength. Most Christmases she returned, showing Dad her publications, her new scars from fieldwork; she was full of stories, shining with intellect, crushing in her accomplishments.

"Compared to you? Of course," I said.

Stupidity had shifted from being an embarrassment to being a defense. Eventually I had learned to like what it did for me. People didn't make demands, didn't expect much. Didn't know who I was. I was much safer that way.

I looked at my sister, my pink, dead sister. "So is everything the aliens told us a lie? Are you really alive in there?" I asked her, speaking to my nightmare. Though I had learned to like the damage she had done me, I still didn't want to thank her for it.

"No," she said, and her eyes lighted from within, violet banishing brown. "No," it said. "She is dead."

"How could you speak in her voice?"

"Her memories are still here," it said.

I covered my mouth with my hands. "What are you Radiants doing? Who are you being inside those bodies?" I whispered past my fingers.

"Whoever we find when we arrive. But away from their homes. We are here to study you, and this is the best way we know."

I lowered my hands slowly.

"You have all her memories and thoughts and

feelings?" I asked after a long time while I tried to sort through my thoughts.

"All that were not overwritten by other thoughts and memories and feelings during her lifetime, or altered by chemistry, medication, or death."

"So you know how she treated me all my life. How could what you did to me possibly mean anything in that context?"

"I know I hurt you."

"It was nothing."

It reached across the picnic table and touched my hand. Its fingers were warm as a mother's touch.

"Don't!" I said, snatching my hand away.

"If it was nothing, why do you fear it still?"

"I don't want you to know me!"

"I know you," it said.

"No one knows me."

It clasped its hands in front of it and looked down at them. Its lowered eyelids hid its radiance; I could be sitting across the table from my sister. "I know you both," it whispered, and raised its lids to stare at me with purple eyes. "I know many of you."

"And we don't know you at all," I said. "How come your skin isn't gray?"

"Because we are shifting to another reality," it said.

"Is this the one where you take over *all* the bodies, living and dead? Are us Earth people totally screwed now?"

"No," it said. "There aren't very many of us, and that's not what we do." It smiled at me. "So many fears . . . We are here to preserve you."

"Preserve us?" I thought of butterflies on pins in boxes with glass tops, of museum displays, static and trapped. Of course, smart light had changed museums a lot. Technoids were still figuring out ways to display things with it.

"To study and remember you, and then to move on."

"You'll be leaving?" Radiants had been part of my life for almost as long as I could remember. What would life be like without them?

"Presently," it said.

"But first you walk around in corpses that look alive."

"A few of us, perhaps. Where we need to make amends."

"I still don't understand that part. You never told me what reparations might involve."

"I looked at you when you did not know how to say no. I offer you a look at me." It held out its hand.

Travel is so easy now because of smart light that I'm not surprised to see people from the other side of the world wandering the streets of Sparrow Creek, though I'm not sure what they find here that isn't easier to get to somewhere else.

The Radiants still relocate, though there are no visible signs that distinguish a Radiant from a living person any longer, except occasional flecks of light in the eyes.

Tony tells me that over time our xenophobia has lessened until it's safe for a Radiant to blend better, but I know this is not so. I listen to him because he likes to be listened to, and I think my own thoughts about Phases Three and Four, how the moment of arrival has the seed of leaving in it because of what you bring with you.

They give us smart light so that we will let them study us, and the smart light changes us until we begin to resemble every other people they have studied and we no longer interest them. Then they move on.

It is strange to know that I, who have lived inside the dim shell of stupidity, could drink smart light—I know now how to do it—and become a Radiant myself.

Here inside my head, I hold a million years of history, a thousand different life forms from as many planets, the memories of a hundred individuals of each life form. I could live forever and not have enough time to examine each one.

I don't know how it all fits inside my skull.

Well, maybe I do. When I look in the mirror now I see faint lavender rings around my irises. Coherent light lives inside me.

The memories I examine most often are Carla's. I never knew she thought I was pretty. I never knew she feared I was smart. I never knew she felt so hollow, small, and scared inside.

That's part of why she checked the alien donor box on her driver's license. She wanted to be useful. She longed to be brilliant.

Now she is part of a being of light.

I won't live long enough to be part of the space-faring race we are destined to become if we follow the pattern of previous peoples the Radiants have contacted. That's all right with me. I've spent all my life within fifty miles of where I was born, and that's where I want to stay.

I can always travel in the comfort of my own head.

JOLENE'S MOTEL

Esther M. Friesner

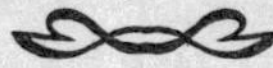

EVERY YEAR WE GET TOGETHER, LAURA AND JOLENE and Trudy and me. The three of us town girls drive up to Jolene's place in the Big Pines together. We tell our husbands that it's the bridge club thing, but that's only part of the truth. We can play bridge in town just as well, and we do, mostly without Jolene. It's just too far a haul for her to drive into town once a week, and besides, she says Mack needs her help around the place. So it's not the bridge. It's the spacemen. If we couldn't talk about them at least this one time a year, I know we'd burst.

We drive up in February, whichever week it is that Mack's got his army reunion. It switches weekends like nobody's business, but it's most always in February. As soon as Jolene finds out when it's going to be, she calls Trudy and Trudy rallies the troops. We usually take my car because it's got the best four-wheel drive, even though my Jimmy says he doesn't know why we need a car like that in the family when his work at Downey's keeps him in town and he doesn't even hunt or fish. He's been swearing to trade it in for something sportier for years. I tell him it's *my* car, so *his* job and *his* hobbies don't signify. Hands off! He starts teasing me about how I only want the car so that whenever his back's turned I can drive up into the mountains to meet my lover. Then I call him an idiot and kiss him and we both laugh loud.

A lot depends on the weather. If we're lucky, the main road's been cleared, in which case any car will do. If we're not, if it's outright snowing, we don't turn back. Like I said, Mack's reunion comes but once a year, and it wouldn't do anyone a bit of good if Jolene was to come into town and miss one of his calls home. Anyway, there's too many ears in town. We like to be alone to talk about the spacemen. We owe them that much.

If it's snowing, the main thing is to make sure one of the girls keeps an eye peeled for the turnoff sign. Even though we know the way, it's easy to miss the road if it's a blowing snow. In a really thick blow, there are times you can miss the sign too, that's how far off the track the Big Pines is.

Mack made the sign himself from a slice of one of the old growth trees. It says Big Pines Lodge, Next Left, but it's no fancy-schmancy lodge. It's just a motel. That doesn't matter to the fishermen and the vacationers. The ones who've stayed there before keep coming back because you can't beat how neat Jolene keeps the place, and the ones who see the sign most likely say, "Wow, kids! A real Montana mountain lodge! Howzabout we stay there?" Except, by the time they've followed that steep, narrow, windy road all the way up and see that it's only a motel, their nerves are too shot and the kids are too cranky for them to turn back without giving the place at least a look-see. Once they see how Jolene keeps things and once they get a whiff of her cooking, they usually stay.

In February there are no vacationers and there are no fishermen, so Mack's declared that month to be vacation time. He's the only one who goes anywhere, though. He has certain thoughts about what needless gallivanting does to a woman. He's the only person I ever heard actually *use* a word like "gallivanting." Jolene says she doesn't mind.

Maybe it would be different if they got the hunting trade, but hunters never have come up this way much either. Laura is of the opinion that they used to, but the spacemen took too many of them and the rest got frightened off. She talks about it as if it's all cold facts, with photographs to back them up, instead of a lot of crazy theorizing. Laura's only lived around here for twelve years, not like Trudy and Jolene and me; we were all born here in Montana, Trudy and Jolene right in town. Trudy finally had enough of hearing Laura's theory about the hunters one year and let her know she thought it was bullshit.

"Jesus Christ, the way you talk about the spacemen, you make them sound like that trigger-happy husband of yours! My Harry says he's the reason the other guys couldn't even bag a rabbit one year, the way he crammed his bag and shot up half the mountain doing it."

It got pretty ugly from there. You couldn't blame Trudy, I guess. Laura'd just been going on about how her little boy, Bill Junior, was so smart that the teachers just didn't know what to do with him, and how it was all thanks to you-know-who. Trudy and Harry don't have any kids, even though they've been married for more than ten years. Trudy says it's because of what happened to her that time they came to choose her. Jolene and I nod and agree with her, right out loud, but Laura never says anything. She just rolls her eyes. It's no wonder Trudy gives her a hard time every chance she gets.

Lucky for all of us that Laura and Trudy always make up their differences. I don't know what I'd do if I didn't have the girls to talk with about the spacemen. If Trudy or Laura got so mad with each other that they dropped out of our group—hey, if even one of them up and quit—that would be the end of it for all of us. It just wouldn't be the same if we couldn't go on together the way we've been doing. They know it. That's why they're as quick to patch things up as they are to rip them open.

We're pretty merry in the car going up to the Big Pines this time. Every year there's something new to tell, something special to share. The three of us who live in town see each other regularly enough, but even so, we've got our secrets. We hold them close, wrap them up in tissue paper, keep them safe for just this once-a-year. It's better than Christmas, because no one else can spoil it for us and we always get just what we want.

Yes, we always do.

Jolene is standing in the doorway of the Big Pines

when we drive up. There's a light snow falling; we had no trouble finding the turnoff or seeing the sign. Everything's soft and quiet, all the world sleeping like a doll in a cotton wool bed. She hugs us tight, one by one, as we cross her threshold. We trade the crisp chill that clings to our parkas and gloves and cheeks for the warm gust of wood smoke and cinnamon and apples that Jolene wears like a bridal veil.

She hustles our coats out of sight while we stand in the lobby—just a fancy name for Jolene's living room. There's a fireplace that crackles with a mix of hardwood and pine, a row of homely old brown teapots on the mantel. They all look alike to me, but Jolene says each one is different.

"Like us," says Trudy. "Because of . . . you know." She can't wait to start talking about it. Every year she's the one who's got the least to say and takes the most time to say it.

It's a sunken living room, the lobby. Jolene says they were all the rage in the fifties. Then she laughs and adds, "But so was I!" We stamp the snow off our boots on the mat, sit on a split log bench just inside the door to pull them off, and pad in our stocking feet past the reception desk, down three steps to take our usual places. All of the furniture is pine, what you could call lodge style even though this place isn't any sort of a lodge, like I said. You'd know it if you saw it. The arms and legs of the chairs and sofa look like someone just chopped off lengths of branch, skinned them, and slapped on a coat of varnish. The cushions are forest green, bark brown, acorn gold, a rough, hard-wearing fabric that's just two steps to the left of being burlap. I'm the first one to notice that there are a couple of new endtables flanking the sofa, two chainsaw-cut sculptures of black bear cubs holding polished planks on their backs.

"Mack went and bought 'em," Jolene says. "He didn't ask me, no surprise. If this place gets any more rustic, I'm gonna puke." And we laugh.

Jolene serves us coffee and sandwiches, tuna fish and egg salad and PB&Js. Trudy asks for plain jelly, like she always does. You would think Jolene would remember, year to year.

"I'm sorry to be a bother, but I just can't eat anything that comes from a, um, vessel of potential intelligence," Trudy says. "They made me promise." She folds her hands in her lap and bows her head over them, like a statue of the Blessed Virgin Mary I once saw in Italy. They told me it was Italy.

"I'm sorry, sweetheart," Jolene says, and she hurries off to the kitchen and comes back with a plain grape jelly sandwich so fast that I sort of wonder if she had it ready out there all the time. Maybe she does remember, year to year, but she doesn't put out the plain jelly sandwich right away, so Trudy can mention her promise herself, all over again. I look at Trudy and see how bright her cheeks are glowing with the pleasure of being noticed. Yeah, Jolene remembers, but Jolene knows.

"I still don't see why you can't eat peanut butter," Laura says around a mouthful of tuna fish. "They told me to give up red meat, except when it'd draw notice to refuse it, but they never said anything against any other food."

Jolene shakes her head and smiles. "I thought we all agreed last year: either they've got a different purpose in mind for each of us or else we might've met different kinds—races—I don't know, but different *somethings* of them. Tribes. Worlds."

For a moment she looks like my mother the last time I saw her. I was only sixteen then, going off to catch the school bus that October morning. She was in our kitchen, sending me off to school. There was flour on her hands; she was making cookies. I still hear her voice calling after me, *Don't be late coming home!* Jolene is old enough to be my mother.

Trudy raises her head and gazes up at the naked beam ceiling. "All I know is *mine* told me they'd be watching. They told me how to live and what to do. They said that they'd be leaving messages with—I remember this part word for word—*vessels of potential intelligence.* They said that included not only all animals, born or unborn, but also legumes. That includes peanuts and beans."

"Like the Pythagoreans," I say. It just slips out. The others look at me. Laura makes a face.

"Ivy, you are just hell on crosswords puzzles," she says. Laura is starting to sound bored. She wants to talk. She's fidgetting with the clasp of her pocketbook and we all know what that means, even if Jolene is the only one who was given the gift of foresight.

Sure enough, the purse snaps open and the photographs come cascading out. Laura acts as if this was all an accident. She lets out a little yipe and starts fluttering over the pictures, trying to scoop them back into her purse. Of course they all slip through her fingers. Trudy looks a little miffed at having her time in the spotlight cut short; she sits on her hands.

I'd play Laura's game, but I've got egg salad all over my fingers.

Thank God for Jolene. She's there to please. She ducks right down to gather up the photographs and say what Laura wants to hear: "Why, honey, is this your little Billy? Just look at how big he's grown! And doesn't he look *smart?*"

"We had him tested," Laura gushes. "We took him to Helena, his teachers *insisted.* They told us he's got a genius IQ. An honest-to-God *genius.*" Her face colors up. "I guess it was worth it, even if it did hurt so bad. My little Billy makes all the pain just a bad memory."

"It shouldn't have hurt," Trudy butts in. "It didn't hurt *me,* not a bit."

"Well, like Jolene said, yours and mine were different." Laura snaps off the words. "Mine *hurt* me." She sounds proud of the pain. She pokes at her hair. It's a nervous tic she's got, always tucking it behind her ears, especially when she's peeved over something.

I remember seeing her in the market when she first came to live in town. Every two steps she'd stop pushing her shopping cart and jab back her hair, one side and the other, sharp and hard, like she was stabbing head lice. Her husband Bill met her in Minneapolis when he was at an insurance agent convention and brought her back here with him. He met her in the hotel restaurant where she was waitressing. Back then, she'd tell anyone who'd listen about how she was only waitressing between modeling jobs. She was saving up enough money to go to New York or L.A., take acting lessons, do some *real* commercials instead of now-and-then fashion shows at local department stores, audition, get a break.

No one wanted to listen. Sure, she was pretty enough to be a model, beautiful, the kind of woman men notice, but as for the rest of her story . . . no one cared. *Coulda-shoulda-woulda* like my son Kevin says. The smartass. The people in this town like what you can hold in your hand and show in the daylight. Any loser can have dreams.

When she vanished from town about eight years ago, I don't need to tell you what they said. Then Bill left too, set out to find her—five whole months the two of them were gone if you add his two to her three—and he brought her back pregnant.

"They held me down," Laura says. "It was all dark and there was an awful smell. I thought I was going to vomit. I tried to move, to struggle, but they—there was leather holding my arms and legs."

"I thought you said there were iron bands," Trudy puts in.

Laura stabs at her hair—left, right—even though there's not a single wisp out of place. "They *felt* hard as iron but they *gave* a little, like leather." Jolene and I exchange a look. This is the way it's always been between those two. When Trudy talks, Laura's just as keen to pounce on any chinks in her story. "And then I felt the surface under me turn wet and ice cold just before they—" Her eyes freeze up, staring back into an old dark place. She clutches the photographs of her son so tight to her breasts she creases a few. She isn't beautiful any more; not with that scar on her cheek, and the way her jaw healed a little out of line.

I am glad my spacemen didn't do all that to me.

Jolene comes and sits next to Laura, puts her arms around her and gives her a hug. "Hush, darling. We agreed we weren't going to talk about the bad parts. You were very brave. And it was worth it. You said so yourself. If you hadn't gone with them—"

"I didn't *go* with them." Laura's eyes are still elsewhere. Her lips are thin and white around the edges where her lipstick missed. "They *took* me. I didn't have any choice. It wasn't my fault. It was dark and I was alone and—"

"It was worth it," Jolene repeats. Her hands—so rough, so red with all the work she does at the Big Pines—close over Laura's. Very gently she picks out one of the photos and holds it where Laura can't help but see it. "Wasn't it?"

Billy's face is the light that leads his mama back from the dark place. The ice that's been spreading over her eyes retreats and she smiles, takes the photo from Jolene and says, "He's going to be something else, my son."

"Mine will too, when it's time." Trudy's voice sounds stiff. Her hands are pressed together in a grip so tight it looks like she's strangling a prayer. "I feel sure that's what they chose me for, only it's not time yet."

"We know," I say. I used to ask her when she thought it *would* be time, but I got my head bitten off for me often enough to drop that. "Don't worry; they'll let you know soon."

She shoots me a poisonous look. Trudy's no fool; she remembers what I used to ask just as well as I do.

She thinks I'm making fun of her. She ought to know better than that. Or she would, if she'd ever really listened to *my* story.

For Trudy and Laura it's not so important to listen as it is to be heard.

"You know they will," Jolene puts in, her voice a healing thing, and Trudy's face slackens, lets go of the hate that's built on envy's bones.

"First I have to hear their message here on Earth," she says. "I have to keep my heart and mind open to receive it. It could come from anywhere. We got a cat two months ago, did I tell you? Just a stray cat that showed up on our porch the day before Christmas. I was going to run it off—I never did get on with cats—when I saw how it was *looking* at me. So I took it in, fed it, got it cleaned up, took it to the vet—"

"You did everything but name it," Laura puts in. "Unless *Get-off-that-you* counts as a name." She giggles. "I saw that cat last time I stopped by your place. And it's a *he*, not an *it*."

Trudy shrugs. "Giving it a name, knowing if it's he or she, that's not the important thing about this cat: it's the way it—*he* looks at me. The way he sticks close to me. I just have a feeling that maybe . . . maybe he's getting ready to speak. Maybe this cat's the vessel they've decided to use when they're ready. They're watching us, you know. They're watching *me*."

Laura shudders. "I couldn't stand that," she says. "Mine came and did what they had to do and were gone. If I thought they were still out there—" Another convulsion of the skin.

Jolene gives her a plate full of lemon cookies. "If they are, they are. It's not our place to question what they want from us. It'll all be for the best."

"That's easy for you to say, Jolene," Trudy snipes back. She really doesn't like to be interrupted. "You weren't given any sort of a trial to bear. You don't have my responsibility."

"You don't think she's got it hard enough?" Laura springs to Jolene's defense. I would do the same, if I thought it was necessary. Jolene wants protecting—she'll never learn to do it for herself—but this is only Trudy. "You saw the marks for yourself often enough! All of those stars, all of those worlds she's got to carry on her skin until they come back—"

"As if they couldn't leave their starmaps carved in stone or etched in metal," Trudy sneers. Sometimes she gets a little crazy, turns envious if any one of us seems to have a better story to tell than she. Sometimes she gets so hungry for attention she forgets how much we need each other. "Why bother burning them into a woman's skin?"

"Why bother making one woman from a jerkwater town their messenger?" I counter quietly. "As if they couldn't find the president of the United States or the Pope or—" I laugh, "or Walter Cronkite!"

Laura and Jolene join in the laughter. I make sure to keep it friendly, not cruel. I don't dare turn Trudy away from us. We need each other. Pretty soon she's laughing too.

"You're right, Ivy, you're right," she says. "And so's Jolene. Just because we've all been chosen doesn't mean the same ones chose us, or for the same reasons. It's not for us to ask. Lord, I ought to know that better than anyone here! When they took me, I was all by myself in that little hunting cabin Harry's got up by the lake, and all I was doing was *asking*. Oh God, the things I was asking! Was it my fault she died? Was it something I ate? Did I forget and take a drink of liquor? Was it maybe that bad cold I had when I was two months on? Did I catch it that week it rained so much, going out to the movies when maybe I should've stayed home like a sensible woman? Was it carelessness, willfulness, plain stupidity that took her from me? I asked Harry, but he just shrugged it away. He said that figuring out if it was my fault we lost her or not wouldn't change the price of apples. The doctor said these things happen, but isn't that what they always say? Was he afraid that if he told me the truth, that it really *was* my fault, that maybe I'd do something even stupider yet?"

Jolene pours coffee into Trudy's clean cup and says, "It's more trouble than it's worth for a doctor to lie to a patient, Trudy. He told you the truth: these things happen. It happened to me once, between our Patricia and Sam, but there was nothing wrong with Sam *or* Martin, when he finally came along."

"Oh, I know that now," Trudy says. She adds cream to her coffee and two teaspoons of sugar. "They told me, when they came. These things happen all the time, and the woman can go on to have healthy children later. So will I, when it's time, when they come back again, when they tell me—"

She's speaking faster and faster. The words are piling into one another like a chain-reaction crash on the highway. (That's how Dad told me mother died. It was the only other thing he'd agree to say to me besides, *Who the hell told you to come back now? You killed her long before she died. Get out of my house and stay out, you whore!*)

There is a little silence. Trudy is pausing to catch her breath. It comes out of her mouth in a long, savoring sigh. Her eyes are full of the starmen, the spacemen who saved her from grief and despair and too many questions. "Thank God they came for me. Harry used to keep a couple of his guns in that cabin . . ." Her voice trails off. She shakes her head, smiling ruefully over what's past. "After, I brought the guns back to town with me and made sure he locked them away with the rest. Can you imagine, a grown man being so careless with guns?"

"You're a smart woman, Trudy," Jolene says. "And a sensible one too."

"*And* I have the peace and the time to listen for the word, when it comes," Trudy adds. "I guess that's one thing the president and the Pope and good old Uncle Walter don't have, the time to really *listen.* They took me into a light that washed over me, inside and out. It was sweet as slipping into a pool of warm water. I came out of it clean. Everything was gone except their purpose—no sorrow, no questions, nothing but what they'd given me to do."

"To wait," says Jolene. "To listen."

Trudy nods, and the bitterness that seams her face lets it smooth into a smile. "When their message comes, I'll be the one free to hear it and bring it to the world." She picks up her coffee cup with her right hand, lays her left hand over her belly. "When I hear their words again, I'll know it's time."

She drinks her coffee. I decide this would be a very bad time to ask her whether coffee beans count as vessels of potential intelligence.

"How about you, Ivy?" Laura asks, leaning over to pat my hand. "Anything?"

It's shorthand for *Anything new?* That's the supposed reason for the four of us to get together: to say whether we've gotten the word, seen the light in the sky, felt the little buzz at the back of the brain that was sent to let us know that they were back. They had to come back. If they didn't come back—if they never even *tried* to contact us again—why then, that could mean that what we told and keep telling each other had happened to us . . . never happened at all.

"Nothing much," I say. "A letter came from my father last week, that's it."

Trudy frowns. "A letter from—? Oh! Oh, *I* see. Well, that's good, isn't it? That must mean he's come around to believing you. That's something."

"Mmm."

I don't tell them that the letter wasn't addressed to me; it came for Kevin. After all the years of trying and trying to make my father believe that my vanishment wasn't my fault, was nothing I'd ever asked for, I was still left banging my fists against a stone wall until they bled. My father has no daughter, but he's willing to admit he has a grandson. Where does he think Kevin sprang from, then? A spaceship? God, I'm so funny sometimes I could cry.

"Well, it *is* something!" Laura insists. "It must mean that they came to him, to your father, and explained what happened. Oh, not as if they came to him the way they came for you—" Laura doesn't want to deprive me of the blessing of being one of the chosen—it might take something away from her too. "I mean the way Jolene still keeps in touch with hers: in dreams."

"Visions." Jolene corrects her quietly. "Not dreams."

Laura isn't really paying attention to Jolene. "Did he say anything in the letter about a dream?"

"Mm-mm," I reply, and take a big bite of my sandwich so I have an excuse to keep quiet until someone else speaks up to fill the void. Someone will. Someone always does.

"I had word," says Jolene. Everyone looks at her; I am forgotten at the same time I am forgiven for having so little new to contribute to the group. (And if Laura and Trudy have only recounted on the same old stories about their alien encounters, it doesn't matter. Over the years they've spun out the familiar tales with just enough variation for cold mutton to pass for spring lamb.)

"When?" Laura demands eagerly.

"How?" Trudy asks, a little skeptical, a little suspicious. She is on guard, jealous of her standing among us as *their* chosen listening post.

As if anyone could ever suspect Jolene! Why, if not for her, I know I would have—but Trudy realizes her error even before Jolene chuckles and says, "Well, not *word,* exactly. Another vision. You know how they come over me, ever since that night I was walking down the road to town and I met them."

Of course we know. How could we avoid knowing? Just as Trudy and Laura manage to retell their sole contact experiences with the spacemen every single time we four get together, so does Jolene. I'm the oddball, not that they pay it much mind. Every space of silence from me is open territory for them to take over, to add to the legends they're making of themselves.

I guess it counts as a legend even if three other women are the only ones that know. They've never told their husbands. I've never told mine. We have our reasons—maybe all different, maybe not so different as we like to think.

For all her smiles and outgoing nature, Jolene's never been one to talk about—well, about things she believes are no one else's business, for whatever reason. Some of it's how she was brought up, I guess, and some of it's simple caution in action. Or fear. But when it comes to the spacemen, she knows it's okay to talk to us.

"This vision I had," she says. "It was so much like the time I met them, at first I thought they'd come back for me. Mack was watching a hockey game on TV. I was out back, checking to see if the animals had been getting into the trash cans. Mack claimed they were, even though I told him that—" She stops, and her eyes stay open but hide things just as much as if someone'd yanked a shade down over them. She's not letting anyone catch the smallest glimpse inside.

"Anyhow, while I was checking the cans, I thought I saw something moving out in the woods, over east. It sounded too . . . too *solid* to be the wind. The pine branches were rustling and snapping, letting something big through. If it wasn't winter, I'd say we had a bear on the prowl. I started toward the sound, like a fool. What if it *was* a bear? They wake up midwinter sometimes—not much, but it's been known to happen—and that's when they're most dangerous. Still, I went closer. I guess Mack didn't marry me for my brains." Her laughter is just a brittle wafer of sound, ready to snap and crumble.

"That's when it hit me, the vision," she says. "It didn't take any time at all, now I look back. I picked up my right foot to take another step toward the crashing sound and there was a flash—that was the vision coming over me—and it was gone before I put my right foot down again."

"Was that all it was?" Laura asks. "Just a flash of light?"

Jolene shakes her head. "Time's different for them, they make it different for us. Inside that flash of light was what they wanted me to see. First there was emptiness, black and cold, like the time I went ice-fishing with Mack and he—well, the ice broke and I went in over my head, all my own fault, Mack's right, I really could stand to lose twenty pounds."

"I don't want to hear about that again, Jolene," I say, and the edge in my voice startles even me.

"Well, ex-*cuse* me." Jolene is so shocked, she lets a little bite and a whole lot of spirit sneak into her voice. But then she recalls who she is, or who she's been told to be, and it all melts away. "I'm sorry, Ivy, I do go on sometimes. I'm a silly woman."

"The vision—?" Laura prompts. "First it was dark, and then—?"

"Oh! Then there were the stars. I was floating out there, not a stitch of clothing on my body, but suddenly I wasn't cold. I could see the bright little sparks burning gold and red and white hot, and their heat was what warmed me. I stretched out my hands to them and they settled down along the length of my arms like little birds. Every one of them that touched me lingered just long enough to flare and die. Even stars die, did you know it? They make a little hissing sound and they're gone. I was crying. I don't know whether it was for the stars or for myself, because they'd been so beautiful and now—"

I know what Jolene was crying for. I could say so, right here, right now, but I won't. Why bother? Jolene herself will say I'm lying, and Trudy and Laura would be too polite to even *think* that maybe I'm right. After all, Jolene's word against mine . . . I've talked to enough stone walls in my time.

So instead I make it a point to put my arms around her and hold her close. It hurts me to do it; she reminds me too much of my mother. Holding her this way, I can't help but remember that I'll never be able to hug my mother again. *Remember?* Hell, it's a sledgehammer, not a memory, and it hits me right between the eyes. I was sixteen when it happened. I was what you call a late bloomer, which meant I still had a lot of that early adolescent obnoxiousness clinging to me. *Hug* my mother? She was lucky to get a civil word out of me, most days. That last morning, when I headed off to school, I don't think I even said good-bye.

And when they let me come back home to her at last, it was too late.

Jolene stops crying. She holds out her arms to show us the marks that the dying stars left burned into her skin. "It's a map," she says, stretching a smile stiffly over her mouth. The marks look fresh and red and angry, two days' old at the most. They must hurt like crazy, but Jolene says they're a star-map that the spacemen have left her to guard for them. This makes her important. It gives purpose to her pain.

I think—I'm almost dead sure that Laura and Trudy know how Jolene really came by those marks. They won't say, though. If they give her the lie, she can do the same right back at them. And if I speak up, she'll still turn on all of us. I can't do that to Trudy and Laura, and I don't see how forcing Jolene to face the truth will do her any real good in the long run. She's been hurt enough.

So I join my voice to Trudy's and Laura's in telling her how special she is, how she'll have the reward for all her faithfulness when the spacemen come back. We praise her for bearing the pain in secret. She needs our words, but she needs our silence more.

We break up our meeting soon after. The snow has stopped; there isn't much accumulation. Jolene walks us out to the car. We're as bad as our husbands make us out to be when it comes to stretching out good-byes. It's while we're still getting in the last few words of encouragement and friendship that Jolene goes tense all of a sudden.

"Did you hear something?" she asks, her eyes shifting uneasily toward the motel.

"Is it them?" Laura demands, clasping Jolene's hands through the open car window.

"No, no, I thought I heard—" She breaks free of Laura's grasp and races back across the snow. The motel door slams behind her. We three in the car exchange perplexed looks, but before we have a chance to discuss what could have possibly possessed Jolene, she's back.

"It was the phone," she says, every word a weight dropped into the void. "I missed it." And she goes inside again without another word.

We drive home in silence. We have no way of knowing whether the missed call was from Mack or not, but we know beyond any shadow of a doubt what will happen if it was. We don't want to think about it. We can't help but think about it. Not talking about it is the best we can do.

I drop off Trudy and Laura at their houses and we arrange for a real meeting of the bridge club next week. I drive home through snowy streets where evening shadows are already stretching themselves out, blue as bruises.

Jimmy and Kevin aren't home, they won't be home until late Sunday. They've gone all the way to the Twin Cities for the weekend. It's time Kevin started looking at colleges, and what's a better time for that than while Mom does her silly bridge club thing all the way up at Jolene's motel? I check the answering machine. There's a loving message from Jimmy waiting for me, a little silly, a little dirty, about what he's going to do to me when he gets home.

I remember how the people talked when I first came to this town. I must've looked like hell; I know I felt like it. After I tried to go home and Dad drove me off, the best I could do was hitchhike west, the few things I owned in this world stuffed in the pack on my back. I wouldn't even have had the pack if it hadn't been a school day when they took me. The ride that brought me as far as this town turned fresh and dumped me here when I wouldn't let him touch me. I sat down right on the curb outside Downey's and started to cry. The people gathered at a distance and stared at me, I could feel their eyes, and I heard someone say how the best thing to do would be stuff me in a car and drive me on to the next town, make me their problem.

I didn't know it then, but that someone was Jimmy. His opinion was I was either a criminal or an addict or just a plain bum.

Then I heard this other voice come in, hard and snappy, no nonsense to it, telling him he ought to be ashamed. That was Jolene, in town to do the shopping while Mack went down to his favorite bar to "tend to business." She lectured Jimmy up, down and sideways, called him a bad Christian, let him know his mama raised him better than this, demanded to know when God almighty had given him some kind of holy vision proving that I was the criminal-addict-bum he painted me. She made him call his mama and his mama took me into their home. The rest worked out just fine, once I came up with a story to explain myself. It didn't involve the spacemen. Later on, when I got a job and settled in and eventually married Jimmy, Jolene told me how she would've taken me in herself, that day, but Mack . . . I told her not to fret over that any more. By then I knew how things were.

I clear the answering machine and stand by the front room window. It's almost full dark and the pane feels nice and cool against my forehead. I think about Jolene. I think I want to see her again, just to make sure she's all right. I won't bother her. She won't even know I'm there.

I go out to my car and grope around under the chassis until I find the spot where I've attached the box. It's about the size of a bar of soap. Even one glance at it's enough to tell that it's made of a metal no one's ever seen before: not here in town, not in Helena, not even in Washington, D.C., nowhere on earth. There are no lines to divide the box's lid from its body, but I know how to touch it just right to make it open. It sighs with the cold air rushing in through the oval gap. I don't know how it works—I don't know how a VCR works either, but I do know how to make it work for me. Sufficient unto the day is the technology thereof. Jolene would tell me not to be so flippant misquoting scripture like that. Jolene believes. I take out two gliders and a pair of hiders and the shot, then I stow the box again.

I don't attach the first glider to the car until I get to the turnoff sign for the Big Pines. The car whispers up the winding road, leaving no tire tracks on the wind-drifted snow. Not from my car this trip, anyhow. There are other tracks, though, a third set crossing over the up-and-back ones we made earlier today. When I see them, my belly slams itself against my spine and my mouth tastes sour. No one goes up to the Big Pines at this time of year except us, and we've been and gone. I know the tracks are going up to the Big Pines, not down to the main road. When Mack goes to his reunion, he takes their only car. What I don't know is how he got back here so fast.

I smack my forehead when I realize that I've been

so upset by the tire tracks, I haven't tagged on the hiders. I fix one to the car beside the glider and the other to me, for later.

I drive right up to where I can see into the lighted living room. There's Mack, red-faced, hollering across the room to where Jolene stands shaking behind the check-in desk. Even at this distance, I can see how her knuckles turn white while her fingers try to dig themselves deep into solid wood.

Yes, I can see everything that's happening in there. My eyes are good, made better by the years of my unchosen exile. When my spacemen finally set me free, they gave me more than the box in parting. They put me back in working order and they even tweaked a few things that hadn't been so good when they took me. All my senses are keen, and if I want to die of cancer I'm going to have to work at it real hard. I don't know whether they did it by way of apology or just plain payment for my time. There never were any explanations between us.

I get out of the car and move right up to the window. I make sure I keep my feet to the path that's been swept clean of snow. I don't have a glider to make me hover over the ground, just a hider; it wouldn't do to leave footprints. I bring my face right up to the glass. If Mack looks this way, he'll see my breath frosting the windowpane but he won't see me.

There's not much danger of Mack looking out the window any time soon, if at all. He's got other things to hold his attention. I can hear what he's yelling, good old Mack: How Jolene's a lying slut; how it's all her fault she makes him so angry with her sly doings, betraying his trust, stabbing him in the back when all he wants to do is love her; how she's the reason for all their troubles; how she's not worth the box to bury her.

He didn't go to his reunion this year after all. He knew she'd be up to something, so he only drove as far as a motel in West Yellowstone and made all his calls home from there. When she didn't answer the phone that one time, he knew. Mack's nobody's fool. He lets her know that you don't have to kick him in the head for him to get the message. He knows what to do about that message too.

And then he's on her. I hug the window, unseen, all-seeing, and I watch as he starts with a slap, another, a third that closes itself into a fist halfway to her face. Blood spatters from her nose and mouth like red raindrops. She tries to run away, which only makes him grab her by the hair and yank her back in range of his fists. When she falls down he kicks her, bellowing how she wouldn't try to escape him if she wasn't guilty as sin.

I have to wait. I don't know how I can do it, but I know I have to. In time the beating stops. Mack's face is redder than ever as he stands over Jolene, redder even than the blood that's streaking her cheeks. His fists are still clenched, his chest heaving for breath. He really ought to watch himself. Everyone in town says that what with his blood pressure and how easy he flies off the handle, his temper's going to be the death of him.

The wide, clean-swept path that took me up to this window is also the path the leads to the front door. I stand beside it, waiting. The shot is very small, a silvery tube about the size of a cigarette, nearly able to fit in the palm of my gloved hand. When they set me down on my own again, they let me know it would protect me. After Dad threw me out, I used it maybe twice on the road, when there wasn't any town nearby or any traffic and the driver I was with forgot the meaning of *no*. Just one touch.

Just one, that's what I learned from watching them use it. They didn't use it all the time—just when the subject was a fully grown man bent on putting up a fight. One touch was enough to leave him stunned. I remember the time they accidentally touched a subject twice with the shot. He almost died; they let him go, though they didn't have to. I think they know something like remorse. I don't think that's something Mack will ever know.

It's a beautiful night. Mack likes to smoke. Maybe he'll come out here to light up, feel the crisp winter air, grin up at the stars as if he owned them too. Maybe he won't. In that case I'll knock at the door.

It's too bad it doesn't leave a mark, the shot, the way his hands have left so many marks on Jolene. I'm going to pretend it does. He's given her a constellation of pain seared into her skin. I'd like to give him a galaxy.

I hear his hand on the doorknob. I press my back against the wall and wait to offer him the stars.

A LAST, LONGING LOOK

James Robert Smith

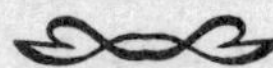

IN THE LITTLE WASHROOM DOWN THE ROAD FROM THE diner, he had stopped washing and was looking down at the hands.

They seemed to be good hands. The fingers were long and fine and one could imagine them holding a camel hair paintbrush, or playing a piano, perhaps. Grime filled the creases and lines in the joints and on the palms, so he had scrubbed and scrubbed with the small bar of yellow soap he had found on the edge of the sink. As he washed them, the thoughts began to collect, the old ones shedding like so much dead skin from a molting snake. Yes, these fingers *had* played the piano often enough in days long gone.

After the hands were clean he had peeled off his shirt and his tattered pants and he had washed the pits of his arms and his crotch, drying himself with wads of rough paper from the dispenser.

Looking at the face in the mirror, he had wanted to shave, although the face looked to have been shaved the day before, most likely. It could use another shave, but he couldn't find a razor or even a knife in the pockets of those tattered black pants or in the breast pocket of the thin coat he had. He had looked at the face, a plain, mild face; it was *his* face, now.

There was some money in the pocket, nine one dollar bills, and there had been two twenties under the lining of the left shoe. So he wasn't without money. He would need a little bit of money when he went to the diner to look at her this one, final time. Oh, he wished he were human.

He felt human, sometimes. The moments were fleeting, then lost. When he was feeling human, he thought that maybe he was cursed, some cursed soul moving from point to point. But, really, he knew better. He just wasn't human. Merely something wishing to be so.

The last time he had felt like a human had been three days before. He had been in the body of a man named Ned Waters. He'd been in Ned's body for months, four long months during which he had used that body and his thirst for humanity to court Ellen Hughes, who he had thought the most beautiful woman he had ever seen. Ned had known Ellen for years, and had never given her much thought until he'd been shunted aside by the new inhabitant of his flesh. After that, it had become Ned's goal to marry Ellen. It had taken long weeks to convince her of that love, as genuine as it had been; Ellen was not a shallow creature. The last time he'd felt like a man was when he had finally gone to bed with Ellen, and she had shared herself with him and they had made love.

In all his years he had found that there were few things so human as love, and the closeness he felt at such moments was among the ultimate human experiences. It was these moments he worked toward. And it was after these moments he was expelled, finding himself outside human walls, drifting again. Drifting until . . .

Until he would find himself peering through different eyes, reaching out with different hands, speaking through a different mouth. This was the way it was. And now, having lost Ellen, having been forced out of his cloak of Ned, he would have a last, longing look at her. He had to. His love for her had made him human, for an instant.

Intentionally, despite the damp night, he had waited in the cover of a long line of shrubs between the road and the peach orchards until the last stragglers at the diner began to vanish one by one. There in the darkness he was invisible to anyone not specifically looking for him, and no one had seen him go to crouch there in the honeysuckle and blackberry tangles. He bided his time and waited, absently picking beggars lice from his pants, pressing out the wrinkles in the dark fabric as the hours ticked by. And he plucked odd leaves and sticks from what he had carefully picked from the wildflower garden untilled by men there on the verge of those tangled shrubs. He plucked and cradled them in his arms.

At last, near midnight, he stood up from his hiding place and peered out. There didn't seem to be anyone in the diner. There was a window of opportunity, he knew, when Victor, who did most of the cooking, would shove off to get home to his wife, who he suspected of cheating on him. There was always about twenty to thirty minutes between the time Victor left and the diner officially closed. Ned usually spent those minutes with Ellen, but Ned had to work late this night and would not arrive until after midnight. This much, he knew, for he had heard the instructions with Ned's own ears. So. He had half an hour, at most.

Avoiding the high weeds that grasped at his shins, he jumped up and bounded out of the bushes and hopped the narrow ditch that held pools of dark, stinking water. He went up the slope to the road and crossed it, seeing Ellen in the diner, seeing her as she rubbed down the counters and peered out from the brightness within. She was looking for the headlights of Ned's pickup truck, and she would not see his form moving through the night, until he approached the front door.

The road was silent and black, blending with the night and the flat sameness of the surrounding country and only the twinkling stars let you know where the horizon lay. He stood there, on the edge of those shadows and waited until Ellen had finished mopping the counter and had retreated into the back of the diner, into the kitchen to begin locking the place down.

Light from the diner fell on him, revealing him as he went to the door and pushed it open, jingling the bell. Going to the counter, he uncradled his arm where he held the bunch of daisies he had plucked from the edge of the orchard, and he placed the carefully groomed stems there on the white surface. And then he quickly took a seat near the big plate glass window, his back to the night so that he could see her face when she saw the daisies.

He sat in the booth that he always used while waiting for Ellen to finish her chores. Most nights, as Ned, he had been right in the same spot, patient as she tidied up and locked down. Right now, he knew, she was latching the single back door that led out to the garbage cans. She had probably put some chicken in a big can for the stray cats that hovered about. Ellen would smell like bacon and her skin feel a bit slick to the touch, a thin sheen of grease from the cooling griddles, but he didn't mind; he never minded.

Ellen appeared from the back and the first thing she saw were the daisies sitting neatly arranged in a fanlike pattern on the white-yellowing-to-brown countertop. Her face broke into a smile, her white teeth revealed, her blue eyes glinting, her light brown hair curly beneath her waitress cap. "Ned?" She started to say his name again and looked around, seeing . . . him. Her smile faded quickly.

He sat, looking at her, his own smile of pain melting at her reaction to his new face. Still, he couldn't blame her. Despite having washed he still looked like the bum he was.

"Oh," she said. "I thought someone else was here. I thought my boyfriend put these here for me."

"No," he said. "Just me."

Ellen put the daisies down, leaving them on the

counter and she fidgeted, trying to decide if she wanted to step out from behind the wood and Formica barrier. She fingered her hair and glanced to the window, looking for headlights. Nothing.

"Do you want something to eat? The grills are off, but we still have sandwiches and pie and coffee." She touched the receipt pad in her apron with her fine hands.

"Some coffee, please," he said.

She went around the counter and got the coffee pot; then he saw her hesitate, as if thinking better of it, and instead she brought him a full carafe and poured him a cup, setting the container on the table for him. "There's cream and sweetener on the table," she told him, nodding at it.

He sat there and looked up at her. He could smell her, now: that familiar smell. The scent aroused him, in every way. "He'll probably just bring you a rose tonight," he said.

"What?" Ellen took a step back.

"He'll probably just bring you a rose. A salmon rose, or just a plain red one if the store was out of salmon."

She backed up a little more. "What do you mean?"

"Ned," he told her. "Ned will just bring you a salmon rose. He's really not all that thoughtful. He doesn't take into account how you might feel on a particular day. So what he'll do is bring you the same flower he gave you on Friday." His hands were busy all the while with the coffee, putting in two sugars and lots of cream. It had been a while since this body had taken in food.

"What are you talking about?" She was all the way

to the counter, now. But she had not turned her back on him.

"Well . . . on Friday morning, Ned brought you a salmon rose, and he brought it to your apartment and left it on the table in your breakfast nook because . . . well, because the sun was getting ready to come up and the light was going to turn the sky a light pink outside your bedroom window, and the first thing you'd see is that color as you opened your eyes. And you'd given Ned a key the week before, he hadn't used it yet, but when you woke up you heard him humming there in the kitchen, you recognized his voice, and when you came out you saw the rose, about the same color as that morning sky. And there was Ned.

"And it was then and there that you decided that you loved him."

Ellen brushed her skirt with her left hand. She often did things like that when she was nervous. She'd done something like it the first time he'd wanted to kiss her. "Who are you," she asked. "What . . . what are you saying?"

"And then the two of you made love. You made love in *your* bed in *your* apartment. Ned loved you." He sat there in his booth and he sipped the coffee, his eyes slitting with pleasure.

"Listen, Mister. You're scaring me and I want you to stop it. I want you to leave." She edged close to the telephone near the register, but still would not turn her back.

"But ever since that morning, Ned really hasn't seemed *quite* the same man, has he? Admit it. How many flowers has he brought you?" He held up his left hand. "Wait. Don't tell me. It's been three days, so he's brought you three flowers . . . and they've all been salmon roses, haven't they?"

"You . . . you don't know me," she said. "You have no business coming in here and talking to me. How do you know my name? How do you know Ned?"

"I *was* Ned." He said it. "I was the one who courted you and made you fall in love. It was *me,* Ellen. It wasn't Ned. Not the Ned who's going through the motions now. It was *me,*" he all but screamed the last.

And then Ellen lost what remained of her courage. She spun and her hands went for the phone. And then *he* stood, she heard his legs hit the tabletop of the booth as often happened with people in a hurry; she heard the cup and saucer clatter against the spoon.

But the silence of the diner was broken by the sound of tires cracking loose gravel onto the blacktop outside, the mutter of a big V-8 bringing a pickup into the parking lot. *It was Ned,* they both thought.

There was a metal creaking as the truck's front door opened, then slammed shut. The front door jingled open and Ned came in. He had a salmon rose in his big right fist and he did not seem to notice that Ellen was upset. *She'd have to tell the oaf.*

Ned went toward her, and she rushed to meet him and it took him a moment to realize she was sobbing. "What's wrong, Ellen? What's wrong," he asked.

Ellen gasped and tried to catch her breath and, finally, she just pointed at *him* sitting there in the the booth where he had sat back once Ned had entered the diner. Ned was a big man. Bigger than most. And he was strong and fast and quick. Any man would think twice before crossing such a man.

Ned's big features turned in the direction of the man sitting in the booth; the dirty bum sitting there and staring blankly at the two of them. He shooed Ellen away, pushed her back with his thick right arm, and he came over to the dirty bum, looming over him. "What's your problem, pal?" *He* would never have said *that.*

The bum looked up at Ellen's lover. Ned's face was big and broad and usually friendly; the kind of face you couldn't hate, not really. The lover's body was strong and quick and younger than the other's. The other knew its strength, that those arms could lift great weights, could hold Ellen's body so easily, as if it were but a feather. And its reflexes were quick: he would see a punch coming *from a mile away* (he might say later, bragging to his pals about the weird guy he decked). So, knowing that body, knowing its strengths and wonderful quickness, he tricked it.

His elbow bumped the coffee pot. It looked just like an accident, the kind of thing a weird little guy nervous in the face of an impending butt-kicking might do. His thin arm jerked up and that elbow bumped that coffee pot. And the lover, his reflexes so quick and his demeanor always on the lookout for friends, reached out, as fast as a cat on a mouse that has finally fled, and he caught that pot that his lover had placed on that table and that the weird guy had just nervously bumped off the table: he doesn't want her to have to clean up the mess.

But the thing is this. While the lover is bent over,

catching that double handful of warmth full of good, black coffee, the weird guy does something. The weird guy reaches over, just an inch or two, really, and he grabs up the great, big, full bottle of ketchup on the table and he brings it down on the head of the fellow with the double handful of coffee pot. There is an awkward silence broken by the big guy grunting, kind of small from so big and graceful a man. The woman gasps. The weird guy jumps up from the table, right up on his chair, and he kicks her lover in the side of the face with his right leg and the power of that kick is spelled out in the way her lover's body goes crashing to the floor like a heavy sack of wet sand.

She can't tell if all the redness is ketchup or blood.

Her lover says nothing, merely lays there heavy and silent with the bright lights overhead glaring down for all to see. But there's really only two of them looking. There's just her. And there's the weird guy.

So she tears her eyes away from the sight of her lover lying there so big and so heavy and so awfully still. And she looks into the eyes of the wiry little man who had come into the diner to stare at her and make her nervous; the strange man who has hurt Ned. She looks at him and sees his eyes. And she screams.

And he knows what she has seen. She has seen the truth. She has seen that *look* in his eyes, that look that her lover once gave her and which he now does not, although everything else is the same about him. This weird little man is looking at her with *that* look and that is what made her scream. That must be what it is, he concludes as she turns to run. Standing on the chair, thinking about what she has seen in his eyes—

all that love glowing out at her—he lets her get to the door and through it, opening it on all of that darkness out there before he jumps off of the chair and begins to chase her.

"Ellen," he yells as he chases her. She is already across the almost empty parking lot. Beyond that there is only the peach orchard and a farmhouse about a mile distant, the lights in its windows glinting in a mocking way through the darkness. The road is cruelly empty of traffic. Ellen has left her purse and the keys to Ned's truck in the diner, and she knows this and hopes only that she can outrun the strange, terrible man.

But he is on her heels, faster and fitter than he looks. Of course, he is a vagrant, used to walking. He has a good wind and she doesn't really have a chance. He has not caught her only because even now, even chasing her down in this orchard, in the night, in the dimness lit only by a crescent moon and the bright stars, even now he enjoys *watching* her, seeing her move, seeing the way her legs push, the way her hips sway. "Ellen," he says through gnashing jaws.

And then he has his thin fingers in her hair and he is not gentle as he clenches down on a great handful of those long, brown, silky strands. *"Stop!"*

They go down in a tangle. His fingers are still gripping her hair and through her panic she feels that pain, feels her hair almost tearing free of her scalp. Her back is to the damp earth, the scent of fallen, rotting peaches all around. He is on top of her, his weight firmly upon her ribcage, one hand in her hair and the other *touching her face.* She tries to scream and he jams the heel of his hand into her mouth, way back so that she cannot bite down and she cannot scream, can only gurgle. "Shut up, Ellen. Please, please don't scream. Listen to me."

There is the sound of them. Both of them panting.

"It's *me,* Ellen. I know you understand. You *have* to. *I'm* the one who made you fall in love. It wasn't *him.* I only used his *body* and now he's going through the motions I set in place. He doesn't even know *why. I'm* the one who loves you." He has to make her see. He has to make her understand so that she will give him that thing that makes him feel like the others, that makes him feel *human.* His free hand caresses her face, touches her chin the way he had the nights he made her love him.

"Remember, Ellen? Remember the way I stroked your face? *He* doesn't do it like that, does he? Not anymore. And." He looks to the sky, then back at the face of this woman he loves so much, who let him feel so wonderful for just that moment before he had been forced out of that body. "And the way I touched you." He lifts himself partially, freeing one knee so that he can reach. "The way I touched you *here.*"

And now, her mouth free, Ellen screams as loud as she can. Even in that house a mile away they will have heard her.

"Leave me alone you *freak.* Let me go. You *freak.*"

He snaps then. It is almost like that moment when he takes love to that ultimate peak. When he has courted and wooed and won that shared moment, when the two join as only true lovers can join. This, then, is the other half, the other way that joins him to *them,* that makes him feel *human.*

The rage builds in his head and flows out of it in an

electric charge that blossoms in his breast and fires down his arms and into his legs and his hands are like claws, like clubs, like knives. Ah. For this moment, for this brief, wonderful moment he is not this alien *thing,* this being apart from all others. In this moment he shares that brutality with them, that red hunger that only they have. For just this instant, as he beats the life out of this woman whom he had loved so grandly, this woman without whom he could not live. He could never continue knowing she was the lover of another. Rage and hatred: nothing else was so human. For an instant he *is* human.

Then, it is over.

Her body is lifeless, that one last breath going out of it, that spark gone. With it, *he* is forced out of this body. He is *flung* out of it. He is ripped out of mortal flesh and he sees everything around them: the trees, the sky, the air, the grass, the dew upon it, the peaches lying rotting in the loam, the bacteria feasting on ripe flesh, the light glittering in the sky. He sees the heavens and wonders for a moment from whence he came, from whence the threat to peace as he leaves behind Ellen's body and her lover lying prone in that diner; leaves behind the derelict man who finds himself crouched over the dead woman he cannot understand killing. In one last glance, he sees police arriving, lights piercing the night. He wonders if the derelict will escape. He thinks (or hopes) that sometimes they do.

Then. He must go. He is being led by a process not completely understood by him. But he is familiar with it. He is tossed far, his *self* coming down to rest.

He opens his eyes and sees himself staring back at his new reflection in the mirror, his hand paused with a razor to shave his handsome face. This time his name is Rick—Rick Collins. *Linda,* he thinks. *You know: Linda is beautiful. I realize that now. I think I'll tell her. Today.*

What a human thought. Love is human.

EVEN SAINTS AND ANGELS

John B. Rosenman

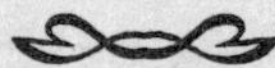

HUBBARD HAD WON $13,000 BEFORE HE STARTED down the steep, swift slope of losing. When the roulette table became unkind to him, he left it for a crap table, and when that, after three bets, made its hostility sufficiently clear, he moved on to one of the numerous blackjack tables that filled the stupendous Las Vegas casino. Which one it was, he didn't know and didn't care. Besides, it made no difference. Whether he was at the Excalibur with its Arthurian theme, the Luxor with its Egyptian, or the MGM with its Wizard of Oz-ian (or, indeed, at one of dozens of other hotels), all the casinos were basically the same: vast, sprawling mazes of glitter, flash, and show, of winking, blinking lights and blaring bells whenever a slot hit a jackpot and quarters started to pour like metal rain.

Sitting down next to a fat, middle-aged woman

wearing rhinestone glasses, he placed a $100 chip before him and watched the dealer smoothly deliver their cards from a plastic shoe. The first time he stayed on seventeen and was beaten by eighteen. The second time he took another card on twelve and went bust with a fat queen.

From then on, it only got worse.

The chips seemed to melt away faster than he could take them from the large plastic cup that bore the hotel's logo. After he'd lost $3,000, he started to wager $300 at a crack, even welcoming the chance to split pairs and double his already healthy bets. It felt as if he were tempting Fate, daring it to hit him on the chin. Unfortunately, Fate was only too happy to oblige. The fat woman beside him ventured only $5 a deal, winning steadily. Occasionally she slipped him an inscrutable look, her rhinestone frames sparkling like diamonds.

Finally, there came a point when he had only $500 left—that and a $5 bill which an excavation of his pockets turned up. Motioning to a waitress, he ordered a scotch on the rocks and watched her head off carrying her tray and his money, her tight little butt twitching.

"Are you in, sir?"

He turned back, seeing that the dealer—a lean man with a pencil-thin mustache—was waiting for him.

Hubbard swallowed and pushed his last five $100 chips into the box before him. "Shoot the works," he said.

To him, it was practically all he had left in the world. But the dealer was unimpressed. The limit at this particular table was $2,000, and there were some tables where the limit went considerably higher. Expressionless, the dealer slid cards out of the shoe to his left, delivering them neatly to each of the four players who sat at the table.

Anxious for his drink, Hubbard watched his cards. A king . . . but what about the bottom card? Lifting it, he saw a black spade—an ace.

Blackjack!

He wanted to shout but managed to restrain himself, only to see the dealer flip over his hole card, revealing a queen above an ace.

It was a push. They'd have to do it again.

At the last moment, something told Hubbard to take his chips and leave the game while he still had something left. Sure, since coming to Vegas he'd lost $4,000, but he'd still have some money to take home! He started to reach for his chips, then hesitated.

"Sir?" the dealer asked.

Hubbard licked his lips. The other players were looking at him oddly. Time seemed to lengthen.

"Let it ride," he said.

The dealer nodded and dealt. Hubbard kept his eyes trained like a spotlight on the few square inches of green felt directly before him. Hole card down, and a jack on top. An excellent chance for a twenty, perhaps even another blackjack! He reached for the bottom card, feeling as if he was going to choke. Please let it be a picture card, a nice queen or a sweet king or a proud jack. Even a ten wouldn't hurt!

Slowly, he turned the card over. A ten, let it be . . .

A king.

He sighed in vast relief. Only then did he raise his eyes to the dealer's cards.

A four of clubs.

When the turn came to him, Hubbard held up his hand to indicate he didn't want another card. Then he watched the dealer nonchalantly flip his own hole card over.

A queen. That made fourteen.

Slipping a card from the shoe, the dealer laid it on top of his cards. Hubbard stared.

The seven of spades.

Numbly, he watched the dealer collect the players' chips and wait briefly for the next bet. The players complied. The dealer's eyes slid to Hubbard.

"Sir?"

His throat worked. "I . . . I'm out."

Numbly, he left his chair and tottered off. Seventeen thousand dollars. Less than an hour ago, he'd had over $17,000, $13,000 more than he'd had when he'd come to Vegas. Seventeen thousand dollars!

Now he had nothing. Not even a dime. At the moment, he couldn't even buy a hamburger at the cheapest restaurant in this hotel. Hell, forget the hamburger. He couldn't even buy a single piece of unchewed gum.

Seventeen thousand dollars.

Now this.

Someone stood in his path. A woman in an Egyptian costume. Nefertiti with a tray.

"Your drink, sir."

He reached out. Lifted the glass on the tray with a trembling hand and left.

"Sir, your change!"

He turned like an inept puppet and clumsily picked up the small collection of bills and coins on the tray. A couple of quarters fell from his fingers and rolled on the casino's opulent carpet.

Expertly, still holding the tray level, the waitress stooped and picked them up.

Hubbard wiped his mouth with the back of his hand. "Keep 'em," he mumbled.

Stricken, he headed off, clutching his worldly goods. Now he could afford a modest meal if he could just find a McDonald's. He tried to laugh, but it died in his gut. Seventeen thousand. Now he had $3 and a few coins.

What should he do now, play the slots?

He stopped and glanced about, seeing row upon row of bright, flashing machines, one-armed bandits whose reels would whirl round and round until the Day of Judgment, long after he himself was dead and oblivious to any pain. Before the slots, players sat as always, mechanically slipping coins in and pulling handles, slipping coins in and pulling handles.

Seeing that he held a drink, Hubbard raised it and gulped till it was empty. His eyes leaked thin tears of regret.

Oh, what a fool. What a stupid fool he was!

He shoved what money he had in his pocket, then stiffened. Wait—he could always use a credit card to get some money and buy more chips. Sure, his luck was bound to change!

He sighed, then set his glass down beside a slot. No. He knew what would happen. He'd only lose again. Instead, he'd use a credit card to get the bare essentials, only what he really needed. A couple hundred, perhaps, just enough to see him through the two days that remained of this convention. When Anson, his boss, had first told him it was being held in Vegas this year, Hubbard had been elated. Bright lights, shows and entertainment! But then he'd remembered the casinos, and his weakness for gambling. For over twenty years, ever since he'd dropped out of college because of poker losses, he had stayed clear of anything that even smelled of betting. Realizing his compulsion, he had avoided temptation. Now . . .

Now he would have to go home and tell Mildred he had lost over $4,000. Either that, or try to conceal the truth from her.

But he knew he couldn't do that. He might occasionally mislead a customer, but misleading *her* was another matter. Between them, honesty had always been important.

Wrapped in self-disgust, he turned and headed for his destination. Even before he was halfway there, though, his face darkened, for he knew that whatever money he obtained, he would only use it to gamble more.

But God help him, he couldn't stop! He had to win back what he'd lost, if only to avoid the hurt look on his wife's face. He just couldn't bear to see her disappointment.

"Hey, Hubby, hit the jackpot yet?"

The greeting came from Chip Fleck, top salesman on the floor for God-knows-how-many straight quarters, the kind of man who could sell a sports car to a quadriplegic. At the moment, Fleck had an arm about a pneumatic blond in a low-cut dress. His free hand held a tall drink.

"Not really," Hubbard said, stopping and forcing himself to smile. "Actually, I've lost a little."

"Oh? Well, not *me.*" Fleck, who had wowed them mightily at today's "Believe You Can Sell" inspirational workshop, produced a thick wad of bills from a pocket and waved them in Hubbard's face. *"Twenty-three hundred smackers,* poor boy. I made my point four straight times shootin' craps!"

Twenty-three hundred dollars? That was chicken-feed! Why, he'd won $13,000, over five times as much as Fleck! But then, Hubbard remembered, he had proceeded to lose every last penny, so he had absolutely nothing to brag about.

He watched Chip Fleck drunkenly pantomine rolling a pair of hot dice and wondered if the man's wife ever suspected his infidelities. That was one thing, Hubbard thought, that *he'd* never do. He loved Mildred far too much to step out on her.

He saw that the blond was gazing at him, a little too long for Fleck's taste. "Easy, Molly Baby," Fleck crooned. "The Master Salesman's the guy with the loot, this honey-tongued *chip* off the ole Devil's block who can sell *anything* to *anybody!* Take it from me, you don't want to waste your time with ole has-been, had-his-day Hubby. Last time Hub ever made Salesman of the Quarter was when he could see his feet and had all his teeth!" He doubled over laughing, spilling part of his drink. The blond shook her head and shrugged at Hubbard.

"Well, I'll see you," Hubbard said. He moved quickly past, ignoring Fleck as he turned to shout something about scrounging up a date so they could all have a party. Continuing on, he drew his wallet from his pocket and extracted his MasterCard. As he did, he saw a long slimy tentacle reach out toward the people at one of the tables, writhing through the air with deadly, pitiless accuracy.

Tentacle?

He stopped and rubbed his eyes. No, there was no tentacle, only a croupier at a roulette table, gathering in the hapless gamblers' losses. He was just imagining things, that's all.

Shrugging it off, he looked up to spot the credit card machine. Then he had a revelation. It was an experience he'd known a handful of times before in his life: a sudden bolt of self-realization that pierced him to the core and stripped him of all his lies. No, he'd never cheat on his wife physically, but he had certainly cheated on her in other ways, hadn't he? Had he told her he'd withdrawn over $4,000 from the account so he could gamble? Or offered to take her to Vegas? He was a phony, and what was worse, half the reason he was gambling now after a twenty-year layoff was to compete with Chip Fleck and other car salesmen who had long since passed him in sales. Whatever he might think of Fleck, he was dead right about one thing. Jack Hubbard *was* a has-been, a salesman whose best days lay in the past. The future belonged to younger, hungrier, wilier men, with sharks who could spot a customer's weakness a mile away. And he had been dumb enough to think he could actually roll back time, win here and show them up! Look what had happened. His losses in college had only been repeated on a much greater scale, and he had nothing but failure to show for it.

But he *had* won $13,000! If he'd just had the sense to quit, to take the money and run! Closing his eyes, he suddenly wanted to do just that, to flee to another world, another realm where he was clean again and spared such insights, such scorching recriminations. But he knew there was no such place, and that eventually he would have to tell Mildred everything.

He stood there gripping his credit card until his guilt and self-loathing faded, and his other motive for gambling returned: not the desire to show Fleck and others up, but simply the need to *play*, to see the next roll of the dice, the next turn of a wheel. Bracing himself, he continued on, looking for the machine that would process his card. Who knows, maybe this time he would win and know when to quit.

Where was the machine?

He put the card away and turned. Odd—the casino looked different, the slots and gambling tables subtly askew, the perspective somehow wrong. Nearby, the section reserved for horse racing reminded him of mirrors in a funhouse, shards endlessly reflecting one another's images in a maze of angles. As he watched, the casino darkened, turned into night. Inching forward, he held out his hands like a blind man. What was happening? How could this be—a power failure? Listening to the sound of his own breathing, he proceeded slowly on, hoping to feel another's touch.

Then he realized there were no other sounds, no rising swell of concern from fellow human throats.

What the hell was happening?

Slowly, it lightened. Long windows appeared and he could see out. He sighed in relief, then froze. Wait a minute, casinos didn't have windows. The one thing they didn't want to remind you of in here was the real world where duties and responsibilities waited. No distractions from the God of Gambling were permitted.

So why were there windows?

Quickly now, the place lightened. Within seconds, he could see his surroundings.

He caught his breath.

He stood in the middle of a vast, vaulted, circular chamber perhaps fifty yards in diameter. Looking up, he saw glittering stars through a sweeping skylight. As if hypnotized, he bathed in their beams for a while, then returned his attention to the room. Gaming tables of various sizes dotted it here and there, and they were surrounded by . . .

Creatures.

He must be dreaming! Turning his head, he saw horns, tusks, scales. Some beings were over twice his height, others he could hold in his hand. A set of tentacles writhed in the air. A snoutlike face swung briefly toward him.

A chill chiseled his spine. His whole body ran with sweat.

He wanted to flee, run back to the casino. But where was it? He could see no doors anywhere in this room! Frantic, he started to retreat toward the circular wall, but to do that, he had to pass some of the creatures.

"Jack, there's no need to be frightened."

He spun, his heart leaping into his throat, part of him wondering who would use his first name.

Before him stood the fat woman with rhinestone glasses who had kept looking at him at the blackjack table.

"What—?"

She smiled. "Do you remember wishing a few minutes ago that you could escape to a place where you didn't have any guilt or shame?" She waved about at the chamber before gently taking his arm. "Well, your wish has been granted."

He blinked. "You must be—"

She patted his arm. "Nuts? No, just consider me a liaison of sorts between the world you left and this one, a citizen of both dimensions." She began to steer him toward a long table about the shape of a crap table.

He started to protest. Was he dreaming? Had losing everything unhinged his mind? Glancing down into her plump, smiling features, he wanted to pinch himself to wake up, only to have her do it for him as if she'd just read his mind.

"See, Jack?" she said, removing her fingers from his arm. "This is just as real as the place you left, only here, there are no regrets."

He opened his mouth, but they were at the long table now. He saw a bearlike creature raise a pair of dice in a huge black claw. Only they weren't dice, he saw, but small, circular objects that glowed like miniature suns. As he (she? it?) cast them onto the table, the menagerie gathered around it followed their progress intently. Hubbard saw the shining orbs roll and roll, bounce endlessly from wall to wall of the table.

Eventually the "suns" stopped rolling, and a clear, deep, unmistakably *alien* voice sang out the result. While the language was not English and he could not even locate the speaker, somehow he understood. "Twenty-four X Triple Prime! Barnard's Star and its attendant planets go to the distinguished Xenabi representative!"

No stickman gathered the objects, collected losing bets and pushed them to the boxman as he would in craps. Indeed, there was no boxman. Somehow, the shining objects simply spiraled through the air and returned to the shooter's claw.

"Establish your wagers, illustrious ones!"

The fat woman gently squeezed Hubbard's arm. "Our visitors come from throughout the cosmos, Jack, and what you see before you is one of our favorite games. Players compete not only for star systems but for galactic clusters—whatever, indeed, takes their fancy." Behind her glittering rhinestone glasses, one eye winked. "Gives a whole new meaning to the term 'high roller,' don't ya think? Now, let's move closer so you can snoop better."

He glanced at the bearlike creature and some of the even more horrifying players. "No! I . . ."

But she steered him forward and as if by magic, the players at the table parted for him. He gazed down into the table's depths, seeing stars and planets and nebulae, endlessly and forever. The universe seemed to open before him.

"Place your wagers, magnificent guests!"

If bets were being placed, Hubbard couldn't see it.

No chips were set in painted boxes. The weird creatures simply stood or in some cases, hovered in the air. How did they gamble—by telepathy? One floating, birdlike *thing* with an immense, transparent eye actually winked at him.

How the shooter knew it was time to throw, Hubbard had no idea. He watched stupified as the bearlike player whipped the tiny suns through the air again. Time after time they caromed off the table's walls in dazzling flight, coming to rest eventually near the opposite end. The players watched closely as if half of creation were at stake.

"Sixty-one Double-Cube Infinity—in the black! The illustrious Xenabi luminary relinquishes the Virgo Cluster!"

Beside him, the fat woman laughed. "Win a little—lose a *lot!* C'mon, Jack, let's visit another game."

Stunned, he let her steer him off. As they walked, he glanced out one of the long windows that girded the chamber, seeing what looked like purple grass and a roiling, golden sky. What was this, another world? Where *was* he? He turned to ask the woman, but they were already at another table.

The next game featured precious gems from throughout the cosmos as prizes. And not merely thousand-carat diamonds and emeralds, but jewels of incomparable beauty for which he had no name. Some had strange, kaleidoscopic images in their cores that stirred subterranean tremors in his mind. A spongelike creature whose sensory organs appeared to be in its middle cast a bundle of ivory sticks on a table with an intricate design. Even after Hubbard's guide briefly explained the game to him, its rules remained opaque.

Other games followed, including one in which players manipulated musical instruments of various shapes in order to win beings from distant worlds. These prizes stood or reclined naked on slowly revolving platforms. As he watched, one player created a haunting melody that won a lightly furred creature with doelike eyes and astonishing sensuality. Despite Hubbard's confusion, he felt the sexual heat throughout his body and started for the table. The fat woman stopped him.

"Your game still awaits us," she said.

"*My* game?"

"Oh yes. It's the only game in town, Jack. A game designed just for *you.*" She eyed him closely. "If you wanted a place where you could gamble as much as you wanted without guilt or consequences, you've found it, love. And here, you'll find that there are no limits whatsoever. You can gamble a million dollars a turn or even more."

"A *million* dollars? You must be mad." He searched his pockets. "All I have is three dollars and . . ."

His voice died. Slowly, he drew two fistfuls of red chips from his pockets. Every one bore the number $1,000 on its surface.

She chuckled and patted his cheek. "I'll hold the rest of your chips for you, sweetie. We'll start you at one million dollars. After that, if you want to go higher . . . well, we'll see."

He gaped at the chips in his hands. "But . . . but what's the catch? Why?"

She winked. "Because your game has a thousand-dollar minimum, that's why. Here, come with me."

She led him to what looked like a human, a man who vaguely resembled Chip Fleck. Boyish and handsome, he greeted Hubbard with a smile.

"Welcome, Jack! I'm your host, and I'm so glad you could join us." He extended a large ruby cup which Hubbard took numbly and placed his chips in. He watched the man motion at a broad, open box before him that was filled with countless, multicolored fibers or filaments that resembled the neural network of a brain.

Hubbard wet his lips. "Is this, uh, *my* game?"

"Absolutely! Indeed, your *brain* was the prototype!" His "host" handed him a glowing, key-shaped object about two feet long with a sharp point at the end. He nodded at the thousands of filaments. "Do you see these? Fifty-one percent are winners and will return the amount you bet if you activate one with this pulser. You understand that all you have to do is speak the amount you wish to wager, and that the minimum is one thousand dollars. There is, of course, no maximum."

Hubbard stared at the man, troubled by the "of course." "What about the other filaments, the forty-nine percent?"

His host shrugged. "If you touch one of them, you will simply forfeit the amount of your wager, plus a memory from your past and subsequent recalls of that memory. Incidently, in all cases, the memory lasts only from a few seconds to a minute or two. No longer. If you lose, it will vanish from your mind and no longer be available to you."

No longer be available to you. Silently, he repeated the words, trying to make sense of them. "I don't understand. How can you take my memories? And why would you want to?"

A shrug. "As for your first question, the process is involved. Suffice it to say that it is perfectly safe. As for the second, there are certain powerful and rather distant clients who collect intense memories from sentient species. Call them connoisseurs of thought, partakers of the psyche."

"And just think," the fat woman said, "the odds here are fifty-one to forty-nine in *your* favor, far better than any house odds on your planet."

"That's correct," his host said smoothly. "Over half these fibers will reward you; less than half will impose a penalty. Try receiving such fair treatment at any casino or gaming establishment back home. You can't lose."

"And speaking of casinos," the woman said, her glasses flashing, "which one in your experience would be so generous as to give you a million dollars just to play?"

Let the buyer beware. There's a sucker born every minute. Cautionary phrases cycled through Hubbard's mind. Why should they *give* him so much money, especially when he was broke to start with? And why would anyone give him better-than-even odds, or want his memories? The last part seemed ghoulish, like the game he'd just witnessed where living beings were the prizes. He looked down at the chips in his cup, then spotted a table beside the woman that was stacked high with different colored chips of varying designs that she was apparently "holding" for him. Looking close, he saw silver ones with pentacles worth $5,000, and golden ones with hieroglyphics worth $10,000.

Hubbard turned back. "Can I cash everything in now and just leave?"

"I'm afraid not," his host chuckled. "You must understand. One million dollars is a good-faith incentive to encourage you to play. It would be poor business for us simply to give it away. However, I guarantee you that any money you win here can be taken back to your home. You'll find that it transfers there with utmost ease."

The woman nudged him. "Why don't you try it first before you decide? Just touch the pulser to one of the filaments."

He looked at the device in his hand.

"Go ahead," the man said. "Take a trial run to see what it's like. There's absolutely no obligation at all to play."

He hesitated, then slowly extended the pulser and touched its point to a red fiber.

Within the complex network, a light flashed from filament to filament in what proved to be a long, random sequence. On, off, on, off, on, off, winking here, blinking there like thoughts in a brain . . .

Finally, the light froze on a blue fiber near the edge. At the same instant, a board behind his host blared and flashed. "That would have been a winner!" the man said. "Go ahead, try another."

Biting his lip, Hubbard touched an amber-colored one this time.

Again the light flashed on and off in a long, unpredictable sequence within the matrix. Finally, it stopped with a filament glowing white near the center. This time the board behind his host was silent and did not flash. Instead, a scene materialized in the air.

Hubbard stiffened, seeing himself at six with a rabbit—his pet rabbit Archie, he suddenly recalled. He watched himself cuddle the animal in his bedroom, murmur childish words of endearment.

Then the scene faded and was gone.

Slowly, Hubbard pointed at the empty space where his memory had been. "If I lose, I have to give up a part of my life in addition to the money?"

"Why not?" his host said. "My friend, the odds *are* in your favor. Besides, you must have *ten billion memories*. Certainly, if you lose, you can afford to dispense with a few. Just ask yourself if you really need them." He eyed Hubbard shrewdly. "I bet you haven't thought of that rabbit in years now, have you?"

To tell the truth, Hubbard thought, it was probably decades. His host was right, why did he need such childhood memories? When had they ever done him any good?

"What's the matter?" the fat woman said. "Don't you think the game's honest? Well, it is, better than Even-Steven. Believe me, Jack, it'll give you a better shake than any game back on Earth."

Oddly, he found he had no doubt it was an honest game and that they would let him take back any money he won here. Still . . .

"What is it, Jack?" his host said. "Surely it can't be any pangs from a useless conscience."

The fat woman smiled and before his eyes,

changed into a beautiful and desirable one, a breathtaking blond. "Nor," she said, "can it be the reluctance you felt earlier about facing your wife with your losses. Jack, there is no guilt or shame here, no mawkish morality or puerile sentiments. Here, the only important thing is to do exactly what *you* want." Raising her hand, she stroked his cheek, exuding a sensual promise. "Look into yourself, honey. Isn't it so?"

He explored his feelings and found that it was. Mildred, his wife, was a frail shadow. What did he owe her or anyone else back in his old life? He laughed, then wondered how he could even think of accepting all this. They put a fortune in his hand, and he found that a fat woman could read his mind. Then, right before his eyes, she turned into the sexiest, most beautiful creature he'd ever seen. How could he just—

"Go ahead," she said, slipping an arm about his waist and leaning close in a wave of perfume. "*Try* it."

He shivered, feeling her soft, full breast against his arm. Before him, his host winked.

"Go ahead, what have you got to lose?"

He gazed down at the half-filled cup in his hand, then at the pulser. "I wager one thousand dollars," he said.

Slowly he extended the device. Should he touch a green filament? No. What about a turquoise one? Frowning, he moved the point here and there. A black one? No, he didn't like the color. What about an orange one?

Yes.

Carefully, he touched the pulser's point to an orange filament, which instantly vanished.

The light winked on and off, on and off, finally stopping on a green filament near the bottom. Instantly, the board behind his host rang and flashed.

He had won!

His host chuckled and dropped a red chip into his cup. The woman, in turn, laughed and kissed his cheek.

"Go ahead," she crooned, "do it again!"

He couldn't pick the same fiber, since it was now gone. But there were plenty of others. A dark blue one—would that start a winning sequence? Or a red one? No, how about a silver!

"I wager another thousand," he said, and touched it.

Again a sequence followed, and again the board lit up. Another winner!

He laughed as another red chip fell musically into his cup, and for the first time turned and kissed the woman. She squealed and returned it passionately.

Let's see. He studied the filaments, the old hunger for gambling rising as never before. Dimly he was aware that his growing lust for the woman only intensified his desire to play, that the two were related, but he was carried on by the rising tide of the moment, by a reckless and growing intoxication. Hell, why bet peanuts? Didn't he have a million dollars? He grinned at the man.

"I wager five thousand."

A touch of the pulser to another filament, and again the board lit up. Seizing a silver chip etched with pentacles from the man, he laughed.

"I wager ten thousand!"

Another winner.

"Twenty thousand!"

And another.

"Forty!"

Again.

He whooped, shaking the cup with its multicolored, multipatterned chips. Then he embraced the woman. Glancing around he saw that his streak had attracted a following. Over a dozen creatures surrounded him now, and more were coming. For some reason they no longer seemed so strange.

Suddenly he had a hunch. His streak was about to end, at least for one time. He didn't know how he knew it, but it paid to be foxy.

Slyly, he bet a thousand dollars and touched a white fiber.

This time, after the sequence, the board was silent. A moment later a scene formed before him, a memory he would lose.

A high school football game was in progress. He saw himself go out for a long pass and outrun his cover, then leap high to receive the pass.

Smack! The ball landed in his hands and he crossed the goal line. Grinning at the roar of the crowd, he started back.

And the scene was gone.

He shook his head. What had he been watching? He couldn't remember.

"Your wager, Jack?" the man said.

Oh yes, the wager. How did he feel? The truth was, he felt great. Somehow he just knew he would win.

"I wager one hundred thousand," he said.

A winner!

"I wager two hundred thousand."

Another!

"I wager half a million."

Again!

The crowd about him swelled, but he had no time for them. In his hand, the pulser thrummed, a wand of miraculous power. Still, he felt suddenly cautious again.

"One thousand dollars," he said, touching a golden filament.

The board was silent and another memory formed—himself as a young man making his first sale. How proud he'd been! Still, did he really need such memories? He had the most desirable woman in creation wrapped about him like a tight suit, and his wand was humming again. Just feel that power!

"One million dollars," he said, touching a magenta fiber.

A blaring, flashing board—another winner! Ho ho ho, he'd just made a cool million! Patting the woman's flank, he prepared to double his bet.

Backward and forward he went, but mostly forward. Somehow, he just knew when he was about to win, and raised his bet each time. Five million, ten . . .

And when the feeling came that he was about to lose, he bet the minimum and watched a memory unfold that soon vanished forever from his mind. But why should he worry? He shook the heavy, almost-filled cup in his hand and glanced at the table on which the rest of his fortune rose in tall, glittering stacks. Why, he must have over a $100,000,000 by now! Drenched in sweat, shouting at every win, he felt a supreme confidence that he couldn't lose. It burned in him, just as the magic wand throbbed victoriously in his hand.

"I wager one hundred million dollars."

Another win!

The crowd grinned and roared, delighted at his good fortune. Whether they had horns or tusks, one head or two, they were all beautiful, especially now that he was approaching the point where he could start thinking in terms of *billions.*

Uh-oh. He was about to lose again. Well, he couldn't win them all.

"One thousand dollars," he said.

And the images formed. Grinning, pleased with himself, he slowly stiffened as he saw what they were. Before him, a young man walked a young woman to the door of her house, where he nervously fidgeted.

It was he as a young man, on his first date with Mildred, his future wife! He saw himself finally find the courage to kiss her, then skip down the walk as she laughed.

His eyes glazed with tears, with the singing freshness of that spring night. It had been the happiest moment of his life.

Then he remembered nothing and knew only that his eyes and cheeks were wet. Trembling, he wiped them with the back of the hand that held his cup. Whatever the memory had been, it must have been something. The important thing, though, was that he felt a new lucky streak coming. He opened his mouth to bet a quarter of a billion dollars.

Wait a minute.

Despite the fever pitch of his excitement, a thought formed. He tried to ignore it, but it came with such force, his head snapped back.

No matter how much he bet, he seemed to keep winning money. Could it be that this game was all an elaborate, devious lie designed to entice him into losing the only things they really wanted? And that would be . . .

He gazed down at the heavy cup in his hand, then at the woman, who stood by the rest of his chips. She smiled seductively, but only reminded him of the tawdry blond who had been with Fleck. He found himself remembering all the phony deals he'd seen, all the slick and empty promises. In twenty years of selling cars, he had waded through swamps of scams and false claims. He had seen cars that stopped running halfway to their new owners' homes, and overpriced lemons with exorbitant interest rates. Some people, like Chip Fleck, delighted in manipulating suckers, in jerking them around until they couldn't see straight. And when he looked at it head on, wasn't that what they had just done to him?

After all, what kind of game was it where you couldn't lose money no matter how hard you tried? Wasn't it a game where what you did lose was the only thing that counted?

Memories. The stuff of his soul.

As had happened earlier in the casino, realization burst upon him. He saw how thoroughly he had been duped, how they had used his weaknesses against him, making him think he was a winner when he was only a colossal fool. This smooth-talking "host" who called him Jack when everyone who knew him called him Hub or Hubby—he wasn't his friend but a consummate con man, an ultimate pit boss who made the ones in Vegas pale into insignificance. And the fabulous woman who clung to his side was an even greater lie.

But the worst thing of all, the very worst, was that he felt he had just lost something far more precious than money. And he couldn't even remember what it was!

"What about it, Jack?" the man grinned. "What do you wager?"

He straightened. "I'm through."

"Through?"

A collective groan sounded, seconded by the woman. She pouted, she protested, she pleaded. She slid her fingers beneath his shirt and caressed his skin.

And his betting fever rose again.

"What do you wager, Jack?" the man said, his eyes shining with greed.

"Yes, honey," the woman purred. *"What?"*

"Bet!" voices shouted. "Don't quit! Play some more!"

"Win, win, win!"

The fever thickened in his blood, lapped at his heart. He felt their wills urge him on and saw the pulser rise in his hand.

"Your wager, Jack," the man said.

He felt his mouth part. "I bet . . ."

"Yes?"

"I bet . . ." They had told him he wouldn't feel anything here. No guilt or shame. But they must have been wrong because he felt them stir again, break through his daze. Even more, though, he felt anger. Anger at how they'd used him. Anger at how, beneath their smiles, they thought he was only a fool.

"Place your wager," the man ordered. *"Now."*

He saw himself reach forward, preparing to touch a fiber. All their wills pressed him relentlessly on, and he knew he could not resist.

Somehow, though, he found the strength to try. Trembling, inch by painful inch, he lowered the pulser with its sharp point. Now it was at his waist, and now his knees. And now he could lay it at last on the thick, plush carpet.

"Jack!" the man said. "What are you—"

"I'm *not* a loser!" he screamed. Rising, he clenched the heavy cup filled with his winnings, and threw them in his host's face. Chips struck the man's forehead and bright smile, scattering everywhere. Hubbard watched a jagged crack appear in the man's smooth face and widen until it was inches across. Inside the braincase, what looked like a white, squirming slug gazed back at him with cold, malevolent eyes.

Hubbard gasped. Despite his revulsion, he thought of reaching into the "man's" skull and ripping the vile thing out. "You . . . you can *keep* your money," he finally shouted, "every damned cent of it. Just give me my memories back, every single one of them. You *can't—buy—me!"*

Blinking, he rubbed his face. What had happened to him? Had he blacked out? Glancing around, he saw the casino, packed with gamblers as it always was, regardless of the day or hour. Slots rang, and he saw that the crowds around the tables were as deep as always.

After a moment he remembered the credit card. Oh yes, he was going to use it to get some money, ostensibly so he could make it through the rest of this trip. Really, though, he had been intending to use it so he could gamble again, try to recover what he'd lost.

He patted his empty pockets and sighed. Well, go get it then.

He took a few steps, then halted, realizing that his clothes had a heavy fragrance. It seemed to be perfume, but even as he smelled it, the scent quickly faded. Puzzled, he shook his head, then realized something else. Funny, he didn't *feel* like gambling. In fact, he felt like he never wanted to gamble again. As far as he was concerned, if he ever saw a gaming table again, it would be far too soon. They could keep their keno and slots, their blackjack and ponies. Though he could not explain it, he knew that gambling was gone from his life forever.

Okay, but at least he needed to get some money to tide him over.

Once more he headed on, though a thought soon slowed his steps. Wasn't there something else he should do first? Something more important? While gambling was a thing of the past, the fact remained that he had lied to his wife, and he sensed that he still had other problems that needed help. It was far past time he talked about them, especially since he knew someone who would listen.

Finding he had reached the machine, he slipped

his credit card into the slot. All right, first he'd get some cash, then head to his room to call Mildred. Pressing a few buttons, he smiled at the memory of a spring night and her lovely, waiting face, and waited for his request for $200 to be processed. How good he felt! It was as if a huge weight had been removed from his heart. He had carried it so long, and now, at last, he was free.

Suddenly a bright star flashed on the machine, making him pull back. What kind of credit card machine was *this?*

Before him, words appeared, scrolling across a screen: You have just subtracted two years from your age. Bet $100.00 for each year younger you wish to be. No limit to amount of bet.

He gasped. What was *happening?* Ignoring the slot which held his money, he gaped at the card, which had emerged from the machine. He started to reach for it, then caught his reflection in a mirror that had just appeared in the machine's center. After a moment, he leaned closer.

Didn't he look younger—his hair a little fuller, his face less lined? Yes, he did!

He turned, glancing about the vast gaming area. He had thought he was *back,* but he was only in another weird casino in another weird realm, wasn't he? Or perhaps it was the same realm. Either way, he was being tempted all over again. And this time, he knew that if he lost, he would grow older and could lose his entire life.

But he didn't have to bet. He could keep his resolution and go to call Mildred! Somehow, he sensed that if he left this casino now, everything would be all right. He would be able to return to his room and call his wife, confess everything.

On the other hand . . .

He removed the card from the slot and stood holding it. Hadn't someone once told him that everyone had a weakness, a temptation he couldn't resist? For each person, it was just a matter of finding the only game in town. If you did, even saints and angels would fall.

He moaned softly and gazed into the mirror. To be young again, with all his life before him! To be given a second chance to avoid the mistakes of the past and reshape his own destiny, a second chance to outwit the Chip Flecks of this world! Who wouldn't do *anything* for that?

He raised the card, then stopped. But what about his resolution to himself, what about calling *Mildred?* And most of all, what if he grew old and lost everything?

He hesitated, his fingers bending the card almost double, bending it so hard, it threatened to snap. Then, bit by bit, his fingers relaxed. "Mildred," he whispered.

Gazing into the mirror, he raised his hand and inserted the card.

A LIGHT IN THE SKY

Christie Golden

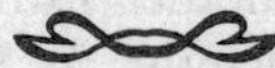

THE LIGHT WAS COOL AS IT BATHED RAY MARTIN'S face. His jaw was slack, his eyes fixed on the source of the illumination. It changed, flickered, danced over his body. He popped the top of another Coors and took a long swig, his eyes never leaving the glowing screen. Like one in a trance, he lifted the remote control.

Seven o'clock. Time for *Sightings.*

"Ray, can you turn that damn thing down?" his wife, Carol, called from upstairs.

Ray's face wrinkled into a frown of discontent, but he obliged, thumbing the button and making Tim White's voice slightly less bone-jarring.

Tonight, Tim informed him, leaning against his newsdesk, *Sightings* would be reporting on statues that wept blood, a pyrokenetic eight year old, and the ghost of some famous founding father's mistress. Ray sighed, crammed some Chex Mix into his mouth and washed it down with more beer. It was acceptable fare. But Ray Martin really watched these shows for information on the UFOs.

Ray watched them all—*Sightings, Unsolved Mysteries, Encounters, The X-Files.* Of course, *The X-Files* was fiction. But it was clear the writers had done their research.

A shadow fell across the sofa, and Ray stiffened. Carol had come downstairs and stood over him, watching him watch the television. Deliberately, Ray helped himself to another fistful of Chex Mix and crunched down defiantly. At least Carol had the courtesy to wait for a commercial.

"Ray," she said, her voice deceptively calm. "Ray, honey, we're not going to be able to get by on what I make at the grocery store for too much longer."

More Coors. No reply.

"I'm working extra shifts as it is. I know you said you needed time after you got laid off but—"

"But what?" Ray turned to look at her. His eyes were hard and Carol, soft and plump and pale and blond, shrank back. "What do you think I'm doing during the day if not goin' out and looking for work?"

It was a lie, and he knew it. And worse, he knew she knew it. He sat at home, his companion the flickering light of the boob tube, and thought about other worlds, ways of life, bright lights in the skies, and gentle beings with long, slim fingers and enormous black eyes. They were the answer, not another futile appointment with unemployment.

Ray Martin was nobody's fool. He knew what was going on. He knew all about the government cover-ups, but no matter what Washington tried to do to people, they couldn't cover up something like this. Not forever. *Chariots of the Gods,* which he'd rented about two months ago, told him that the aliens had been here before and done wonderful things. There were increased reports of, well, sightings and encounters, some of them scary, some of them beautiful. Ray knew in his bones that soon, soon, they would come for him. And he'd finally be able to know just what kind of a paradise they were offering mankind.

Who needed a damn job when the UFOs were about to change the world?

But he couldn't explain this to Carol. He'd tried to get her to watch these shows with him, but she simply didn't understand. She scoffed at the Mars face, calling it a freak geological formation. She ignored all the evidence of the crash at Roswell, and when he had dragged her down for a day trip to the International UFO Museum and Research Center in Roswell she had mortified him by laughing at the displays. The strange lettering that a very credible witness had reported seeing on a broken metal spar was "ridiculous." The little two-foot-high, silver-bodied, black-eyed alien statue that welcomed visitors was "dumb." The most believable thing in the museum, Carol had said on the way back, was the dummy alien from the movie *Roswell,* on permanent loan.

As they were leaving, Carol had pointed at a car

parked near the museum—probably the car of one of the helpful, elderly women who worked there. Some cruel kid had traced an alien face in the dust on the backseat window along with the words "Abduct us!"

"Maybe you should do that to our car, Ray!" she had laughed.

Ray wasn't laughing. He had gotten very angry at Carol and refused to speak to her the entire trip back to Colorado. At night, he turned his back to her, ignoring her tentative overtures, until she finally stopped making them. They barely spoke to one another these days, except when she nagged him to get a job.

Which she was doing again right now.

"We've only got a couple hundred in the bank now, and—"

"Back on." His voice was hard, brooking no argument. He stared at Tim White, crisp, clean, and convincing as he chattered about little Amy McDonald, who seemed to have a genuine ability to set things on fire with the power of her mind.

For a moment, Carol sat silently by her husband's side. Then she rose, just as quietly, and went upstairs.

Ray settled back into his La-Z-Boy recliner. That was better.

"So, you seen any UFOs yet?" cracked Jimmy DiMarco as Ray got in the Honda and slammed the door.

Ray stared down at his bowling ball, on the mat between his feet. "No, but there are reports all the time. You just wait, Jimmy. Any day now someone's gonna get some hard evidence and you scoffers are gonna have to believe it. And then you'll know all along I was right."

"I'll believe it when I see 'em," laughed Jimmy. Jimmy was about ten years younger than Ray, but they had bonded instantly the day they had met, at Bowled Over bowling alley over on Colfax. Jimmy was new to the team that year, but had helped them get a few tantalizing steps closer to victory. That had been back in '89. Seven years later, they were best buddies, whether it was cheering each other on at the bowling alley, quaffing a few beers at a local bar afterward, or staring silently, in deep masculine communion, at the tube during football season.

Ray couldn't blame Jimmy. He didn't watch *Sightings* or *Encounters*. He didn't know what it felt like to watch ordinary people, very credible, honest Joes and Janes, telling stories that were beyond belief—almost. These people were sincere. He'd scoffed too, once. But you couldn't just deny the facts. Some of these people lost everything when they spoke about their abduction—families, jobs, reputations. Now why in hell would someone risk everything for a lie, and a lie that was sure to not be believed? Didn't make sense, and everything in Ray Martin's world had been clipped, squeezed, trimmed, and adjusted so that it made sense.

Maybe a few of these people were indeed liars or jokesters. Maybe a few made a couple of bucks off their stories. But most of the abductees had frightened looks to their eyes, a wariness, and a sincerity that Ray believed utterly.

Only one thing was wrong. Most of these people talked like the aliens were bad—taking samples, hurting them, conducting obscene experiments. They spoke of terror and fear. Ray thought otherwise. He knew, deep in his gut, that the aliens weren't coming here just to hurt people. They wanted to help. They weren't evil—they were good, but people just didn't know enough yet about them to realize it. Maybe the folks the aliens performed "experiments" on were getting vaccines or something. Nobody'd ever thought about *that* when they went on *Encounters*. Maybe they were helping humanity—strange, silent, ethereal alien visitors doing what they could to help the people of Earth.

Yeah. That had to be it. Had to.

Jimmy changed the subject and soon both men were laughing at a fellow team member who was so henpecked he barely stood up straight anymore.

The phone rang, shrilling in Ray's ear like the alarm siren from a UFO in trouble.

Blinking, his heart thudding with alarm, he fumbled for the phone. The clock by his bed showed 5:02 in bright red letters.

" 'Lo?" he rasped.

Silence, but someone was clearly on the other line.

"Who the hell is this?" growled Ray, propping himself up on his elbow. Was Carol, damn the bitch, having an affair behind his back?

"Ray." The word was a whisper. "Ray. I . . ." the caller began to cry.

Fully awake now, Ray sat upright. "Jimmy? That you?"

More sobs. "Ray, I . . . oh, God, God, you were right!" Now Jimmy's voice was lost in uncontrollable crying.

"Right about what?" Ray rubbed at his eyes. Jimmy wasn't usually a drinking man. Hell, he could knock back a six-pack with the best of them, but Ray'd never seen Jimmy reduced to a sobbing drunk.

"Them!" A hitch in the breath. "Them, Ray. They . . . they were here . . . and they took me . . . oh, my God, my God . . ."

Ray's heart did a flipflop, then began to slam against his chest as if it were trying to break out.

"The . . . aliens? Jimmy, did you see a UFO?"

"Oh, good Lord," groaned Carol. She rolled over and wrapped the pillow around her ears.

Ray ignored her. "Jimmy, listen. Listen! Get a grip, okay? Better. Now, tell me what happened."

"Nobody will believe me—"

"Ain't true. I believe you and I can tell you who to talk to who'll believe you too. Okay? Tell me."

Oh, God. God, was he excited. The hair all over his body stood on end, tingling with anticipation.

Jimmy gulped, then began. "Well, earlier tonight, I fell asleep like usual. Then this light came flooding in to the window. Damn, it was like sunlight—like a floodlight—brighter. Woke me up. But I couldn't move a goddamn muscle. I just lay there on my back, staring. And then—"

"Go on." Sweat gleamed on Ray's brow. His hand hurt and he glanced down absently to see that he'd been clutching the sheets with a death grip.

"They were in the room, and they took me, and—"

"What did they look like?"

"Christ, Ray! Everyone was right! All of you sons of bitches were right! They looked like that damn *Close Encounters* movie! Tall, and gray, and these big black eyes and fingers. Oh, God, their fingers . . . "

Ray's vision suddenly blurred. Something warm and wet coursed down his cheeks. He realized that he was crying. Not sobbing, like Jimmy, simply, quietly, weeping tears of joy.

He believed Jimmy. Jimmy would never call him like this unless he was convinced that what had happened to him was no nightmare nor drunken hallucination. Oh, yes, he'd been right. He'd been right. He listened, wiping his unshaven face with a big, meaty hand now and then as the tears kept coming. He listened to Jimmy spill forth a story of being taken aboard a ship, poked and probed and analyzed by strange beings with luminous faces and big black eyes. A story that could have come right out of *Encounters*.

A story that Ray Martin would have given his life to have experienced.

At last, Jimmy wound down. Then he said something completely unexpected.

"I want you to come over tomorrow night with your gun, Ray. I want you to blow one of those things to kingdom come. I want to have a body to take to the newspapers and blow the goddamn lid off the goddamn government coverup."

"Jimmy, I—I—" Ray didn't want to shoot the aliens. He wanted to be taken away by them; away from this squalid world of child molesters and government coverups and fat wives and a demeaning search for a demeaning job that paid a paltry amount of money. Damn it, where was the justice? Why did they come for Jimmy and not for him?

"Okay, Jimmy. I'll be there for you. You won't get taken by them again. I swear to God."

Ray barely recognized Jimmy as his friend opened the door to his small one-bedroom house. He looked as if he'd aged a decade. His face, pale and haggard, trembled into a smile as he admitted Ray, holding open the screen door for him. There were gray streaks in the thick black hair that Ray was willing to bet hadn't been there twenty-four hours earlier.

"Christ, Jimmy," was all he could think of to say. "Christ."

"Yeah," rasped Jimmy. "I look like hell and don't I know it." He raised a hand that jittered and rubbed it over his stubbled chin. "Want some coffee? I been making pot after pot today." He smiled without humor. "Better than cracking open a bottle, I figure."

Ray nodded and stepped into the cramped kitchen as Jimmy reached for a clean cup. "Thanks for bringing the gun," said Jimmy, not meeting Ray's eyes.

"No problem." Ray propped the aforementioned weapon up against the wall and accepted the steaming cup of coffee.

"Ray . . ." Jimmy sat down heavily on the cheap chair, propped his elbow up on the formica table. "Ray, I don't know how to tell you how sorry I am. You know—that I thought you were full of it."

Ray gingerly sipped at the hot coffee. It tasted terrible, but by God it was strong. He sat down himself.

"Ah, don't worry about it." He nodded over at the rifle. "We're gonna get us some solid evidence tonight, and then no one's gonna laugh at us."

Jimmy nodded, his dark eyes distant, unfocused. Then, to Ray's shock and horror, those eyes filled with tears and Jimmy began to sob.

Uncomfortable, Ray sat, his big hands clasped about his hot mug. He couldn't think of anything to say, to do, and so he simply waited until Jimmy had cried himself out. Several long, awkward minutes later, the younger man's rasping sobs mutated into soft whimpers, and Jimmy wiped at his wet eyes. He rose and went to the fridge, returning with a six-pack of Bud.

"To hell with it," he said, wrestling free a can, popping it open and taking a long, thirsty drink.

Ray kept to the coffee. He didn't want to risk ruining his aim—not tonight of all nights.

The evening crept by. Finally, around nine o'clock, Jimmy rose. "It was eleven when I went to bed last night. Maybe if I—we—get there earlier, they'll come sooner. Goddamn it but this is . . ." There were clearly no words, for Jimmy turned and led the way up his rickety stairs to his bedroom.

Clutching the rifle like a lifeline, Ray followed.

The bedroom was exactly what Ray would have expected a bachelor's room to be—chaotic. It was, he mused with a hint of wistfulness, what his own room used to look like before he married Carol and she picked up every damn little thing. Ray brushed a several-day-old pile of clothes from off the one old, lumpy chair and sat down while Jimmy threw himself onto the unmade, slightly stained bed. He added to Ray's discomfort by immediately curling up into a fetal position, as if he couldn't help it.

"Turn the light off, Ray," came Jimmy's voice, hollow, thin, nothing like the robust Italian bellow that used to issue from the man's throat. "They might come sooner if they think I'm asleep," he added, repeating himself.

"Let me load this baby first," said Ray. He busied himself with putting bullets in the gun, the oft-practiced ritual calming him, making his hands steady. When he was a boy, he'd shot targets and bottles and squirrels. Later, his daddy had taken him to shoot duck and deer. Sometimes he'd aimed the rifle at a fox or coyote or two. But never, not in his entire life, had he lifted the rifle and stared down its sight at the prey he would claim tonight.

He finished his task, reached up and snapped off the light. The blinds were not closed, and Ray stared out of the windows at the street below and houses across that street. It was dark, but streetlights provided some yellowish illumination. Somewhere, a dog barked and someone yelled at it. A car pulled into the driveway of Jimmy's neighbor and a fat, balding man heaved his bulk out of the too-small car and lumbered toward the door.

The very ordinariness of the scene thrilled Ray as he sat, watching like a voyeur, his hands absently stroking the cool metal of the gun. Those people would eat dinner, watch TV, maybe fight with, maybe make love to their spouses, go to sleep, and wake up the next morning to do it all over again. Whereas he, Raymond Martin, would never be the same. He was fundamentally different from these people he watched with a strange, condescending eye. He was different even from Jimmy, who had had the great good fortune to be carried away and returned by the strange beings who rode the unidentified flying objects that most saw only as strange lights in the sky. Jimmy was afraid, lay even now curled up like a goddamned shrimp in his bed. But Ray knew on a deep level what these beings were; knew, and waited for their eventual arrival with a throb of joy.

The hours passed.

And unbelievably, at some point in the darkness, Raymond heard a deep, rumbling sound that meant that Jimmy had gone to sleep.

Maybe that was all right. Maybe the aliens needed to know that their target was asleep before they would come. That did not mean that Ray would be able to catch a wink, however.

Eleven.

Midnight.

One.

Ray's eyes were growing heavy. The initial excitement had subsided in the face of hours of sitting quietly with nothing to do. He yawned, and lifted his hands to knuckle his eyes.

At that moment, the light came, with the suddenness and power of a chord at the opening of an overture. One second the room was dim, lit only by the faint illumination of the streetlights; the next it was blindingly bright. Pain jolted Ray's eyes as he cried out, using his hands to shield himself from that unbearable brightness.

Fear sang through him as that light fell upon him. It was as if its brilliance threw light even on his darkest inner thoughts, as if nothing were secret and sacred. But then, Ray had known that he could hide nothing from the aliens anyway.

Still Jimmy slept on.

Ray's eyes adjusted, though he still had to squint to see. He thought he heard a faint humming sound, but it might have just been in his own head. And as suddenly as the light from their space-faring vessel had appeared, so did the otherworldly travelers themselves.

Three of them stood beside Ray's bed, one on each side and a third at the foot. The humming, a sound as sweet and bright and overwhelming as the light, rose and permeated Ray's body.

He began to weep; not loud, hoarse, unmanly sobs like Jimmy had uttered earlier, but silently, just as he had when Jimmy had first called him. The tears filled his eyes, made their way softly down his cheeks, and kept on coming. He was no more able to stop the tears than he was to dim the light or silence the sound. He knew somehow that this, too, was part of the experience of witnessing the aliens at long last.

They were exactly as he had imagined, sketched, dreamed them. Tall, taller than he, slim, delicate as a butterfly but, he knew, stronger than an elephant. As he watched, caught in the moment like a fly in amber, they reached long, thin, four-fingered hands to Jimmy and caressed the sleeping man's brow. Dear God, such gentleness, such care in those touches. Words like music, but spoken for the mind and not the ear, passed between them and were overheard by Ray.

As one, with the grace of a dancer in an exquisitely choreographed ballet, they leaned forward, ever so gently slipping their arms beneath the body of the sleeping man.

Giving Ray the clear shot he wanted.

There was not a hint of trembling in his arms now. He knew exactly what he was doing, felt calmness descend like something physical as he lifted the rifle, lined up the shot, and squeezed the trigger.

The crack of the rifle shattered the lulling hum of the aliens' mental speech. They jerked backward, startled, and stared down at the ruin of a man on the bed.

There was not much left of Jimmy's head. Blood, shards of bone and bits of brain splattered the bed, headboard, and the three aliens who fluttered and hummed anxiously.

Perfect, Ray thought to himself.

He stood on legs suddenly gone rubbery, still clutching the rifle.

"He didn't want you," rasped Ray. His voice sounded thick and dull in his own ears; nothing like the beautiful, wordless communication of the aliens who now, finally, turned their attention upon him. "He was afraid. He didn't want to go."

He gestured frantically, pointing at his chest. *"I*

want to go! He's dead, he's of no use to you now. Take me. God, please, please, *take me!*"

His voice rose and shattered on the last word. Tears again filled his eyes and his legs refused to support him. Ray stumbled, then fell to his knees, keeping his gaze locked with the huge, unreadable, black, cat-shaped eyes of the aliens. He put the rifle down and extended his hands in an ancient gesture of pleading—a gesture so old that he was sure the aliens must have seen it, have known it, when they first saw it in Rome or Athens or Jerusalem or in the jungles of Peru or on the plains of Africa . . .

The three aliens, again moving as one, turned to commune among themselves. Jimmy's blood and brains still clung to their—skin? space suits? Ray didn't, couldn't know—but then they turned toward him.

Their expressions had never changed. But something else, something very important, had, and Ray felt terror clutch at his gut. Dimly, he heard the wail of approaching sirens.

"No," he whispered. "No, please . . . please, I killed my best friend for you . . ."

The middle alien moved now, his fellows closing ranks behind him. He reached out a hand, long, slender, floating like a bit of a spider's web caught in a playful breeze, and placed cool fingers on Ray's head.

And the words came. The words that were never spoken, but merely sensed. The words that echoed in Ray Martin's tortured soul like the damnation of a loving god. The sirens grew louder. They were almost here, almost here, but Ray didn't care. He was too busy crying silently for the dreadful thing the alien was doing to him.

Your violence has sealed your fate. We could not take you now even if we wished, came the words. And then, the worst punishment of all:

Forget.

ALIEN AND FUGUE

Lois Tilton

MARTIN VANCLEVE HANDED HIS ID TO THE GUARD AT the last checkpoint. Master Sergeant Kovic displayed no sign of recognition while he put the card through the scanner, nothing to indicate that he'd ever checked Vancleve through this point before. It was all procedure with Kovic.

Following procedure, Vancleve submitted to the personal scan, yielding a speck of his tissue so that its DNA could be compared to the sample in the security database. At last the sergeant handed the card back. "Clear to pass through, sir."

Kovic's glance followed him toward the locked door beyond the checkpoint, where procedure didn't authorize him to pass. The sergeant had never seen the being he guarded, and it wasn't his job to wonder what Vancleve was doing once he was past this point. Four years ago, there'd been a continual traffic of interrogators and guards through the checkpoint, but things were different now, and official interest in the alien had diminished since that first, urgent year. Now Vancleve was the most frequent visitor, yet the security procedures hadn't changed, even though Kovic had checked him through at least three times a week for more than a year.

Someone in authority, most likely Colonel Cho, had decided that the alien prisoner shouldn't be left in complete isolation while there was no interrogation underway.

How do we know that he's not insane, after all this time?

Would you still be sane?

Vancleve paused in front of the door, then turned aside to switch on a wall monitor. The screen showed a figure crouched on the floor, too many long limbs and impossible angles: alien.

And by now, almost as familiar to Vancleve as his own face in the mirror.

Standing in the stiff new uniform, Vancleve tried not to let his attention stray to the blank monitor screen instead of the UNEarth general addressing him. "Captain"—he was Captain now, no longer Doctor—"you've already signed the Secrecy Act, you understand that you're now subject to military discipline. In light of these facts, I will repeat: what you're about to see here will *not* be discussed with anyone outside this facility."

It wasn't the general's tone that kept Vancleve's eyes from glancing to the monitor, it was the look on the face of the man standing beside him, the man in the colonel's uniform. No mercy in it. But Vancleve kncw what he was about to see. The enormity of it frightened, thrilled him.

As the picture flashed onto the screen above the general's head, he leaned forward, unconsciously holding his breath. Beyond a doubt: *alien.*

"Your task . . ." The general was addressing him again, and he had to force a part of his attention back away from the screen, "will be to help establish communication with this being. As quickly as possible. Using any means necessary."

He used his key and the door slid open. The alien looked up from where he **(He? Does it make any sense to use our gender terms?)** knelt on the floor of the cell. The eyes, oversized in the wedge-shaped head, irised into focus, and the alien raised himself up from the floor with a long-limbed, almost spiderish motion.

"Hello, Zhrrrch."

Over a year just to get a name out of him!

If that really is his name. If they even have names.

It was five years now since this sole survivor of an unknown race had been pulled from the wreckage of his ship, a ship that had fired on an armed UNEarth probe, in the outer reaches of the Oort Cloud. Nearly four years since the interrogators' team had been confronted with their subject, in God-only-knew-what mental state after the transit to Earth Mainbase, confined in isolation all that time.

Establish communication.

As quickly as possible.

Any means necessary.

The team had only trial and error to guide them, since it was too risky to submit the alien biochemistry to the drugs that extracted the truth from human subjects. They were back, as Ramachandra said, to the days of the rack and thumbscrews. Which remark Vancleve considered too close to the truth for humor. But the situation was urgent, they all understood that.

How much more of this?

He can't keep it up forever. Sooner or later, he'll crack, he'll have to talk.

But what if he never does understand us?

What if he's telling us what we want to know, but we can't understand him?

"Hello, Zhrrrch." The name—what they took to be his name—was a high-pitched whistle. Vancleve always tried to produce the best approximation of the sound that a human voice was capable of. Most of the others simply relied on the computer's translation module, but Vancleve considered it important to make the effort.

In his own mind, he thought of the alien as Ric.

The alien replied with wary politeness: *Khvvv*. The sound emerged as a low buzz, but Vancleve's link obligingly rendered it as his name. Ric could recognize the various members of the team, distinguish them as individuals. His eyes always blinked more rapidly whenever Colonel Cho was present, which the computer interpreted as a sign of apprehension.

Vancleve knelt, which the computer analysis had

suggested as a low-threat posture. After a moment, Ric settled to join him.

Someone in authority had noticed recently that the alien seemed to trust Vancleve more than any of the other officers in the interrogation team. This was a factor that could be used.

Vancleve wasn't looking forward to what he was going to do, but he had his orders. "The leaders of Earth have decided to send a major expedition back into the Oort Cloud. The zone where we met your ship. Do you understand? Many ships—a war fleet. If they find more of your ships . . . well, then we don't know what will happen. We don't want to fight your people. We don't want war. But we have to know if they will attack us again. Will they negotiate, talk with us? Will they believe us if we tell them we want peace?"

And what does that word mean to him: "peace"? What does he hear when the computer makes that sound?

"I don't know."

"I don't know."

Always the same answer, always the same, no matter what they tried. They could establish communication, they could force the alien to speak, but never to reveal anything they wanted to know.

What if he really doesn't understand? What if it's a fault in the algorithm and the computer's feeding him garbage? Feeding it back to us?

What if he really doesn't know?

"How far away is your homeworld, Zhrrrch? What are the navigation coordinates?

"What was your ship doing so close to our solar system? Why did you come here? Did you know this system was populated? Did you know we were here?

"Why did your ship open fire?"

"I don't know."

He could be telling the truth. Maybe he really doesn't know.

He could be following orders not to talk.

What if he never does? How long do we keep this up?

How long can he keep this up?

"Are you refusing to speak? Is that it?"

"I know nothing."

With some urgency now, Vancleve pleaded, "Ric, there isn't much time left! Soon, in a few weeks, it may be too late. The fleet will be on its way. It isn't only human lives that might be lost. Some of your own people might be killed. Can't you say anything to help us?"

"I know nothing to say."

Vancleve took a breath. "You could go, you know. With the fleet. Possibly back to your own people, if we find them out there. You could get out of this place! All you have to do is cooperate," he urged. "Give us a reason to trust you. Do you realize how long it could be before you get another chance? It's been five years already! How long do you want to stay here? Locked up alone in this room?"

The alien's eyes blinked rapidly, a sign of distress. But he wouldn't speak.

He'll talk. It's just a matter of time.

God, how long, though? How much more?

Vancleve wondered if Ric knew he was lying. UNEarth Command had considered the option of bringing the prisoner along on the expedition to seek out signs of more alien ships, but the decision had been negative. The alien wasn't considered reliable. And Vancleve supposed they couldn't risk the consequences if Ric's people learned what had been done to him.

"I know nothing."

The message was waiting on his desk screen: My office. Cho.

A muscle in Vancleve's belly twitched in nervous apprehension. What did the colonel want now?

"Sit down, Captain."

Vancleve did, stiff-backed at the edge of the chair facing Cho's desk. The colonel's face was smooth and ageless, and it revealed nothing of the man's feelings. "You're aware that Command has moved up the schedule for the fleet's departure."

"Yes, sir. On the fifth of April."

"Less than two months." Less than two months to get results. "I suppose you know about the alien spool player?"

"I've studied the file."

The alien ship had fired first, then self-destructed almost as soon as the UNEarth vessel returned the attack. The investigators probing the wreckage had been meticulously thorough. All the data in its navigation system, in its computers, had been obliterated. But the destruction had been incomplete, and among the objects recovered, besides the single living prisoner, was an item eventually identified as a spool player, in a case complete with cylinders recorded with some kind of alien data—or was it speech? Or was it music?

To Vancleve, who'd listened to the sample included with the file on the object, it sounded like music.

But even so, the spools could still hold information, couldn't they? Encoded in musical form?

"Do you have an opinion about the spools, Captain?"

"No, sir, I don't, really. Except that, from the little I've heard, I agree with the analysis—those aren't alien voices on the recording." But of course it was only a copy that he'd listened to, and he knew that the alien recordings ranged upward into frequencies beyond the capacity of the human ear to follow, as did the sounds of the aliens' speech.

It was a tonal language, that had been easy to determine—like Chinese, only much more so, as if there were no distinction between speech and song. But although the translation team managed to produce a translation algorithm for the alien prisoner's speech, they'd never succeeded in decoding the message on the spools. If there were any message.

UNEarth Command still guarded them jealously, convinced by their own desires that somehow the spools must hold navigation data, a key to the location of the alien homeworld, some valuable secret. So Vancleve could hardly believe it when Cho unlocked a cabinet behind his desk and took out a familiar-looking case. "Here. Take it. Give it to him. I want to see what he does with it."

Wondering, he found a latch, popped the case

open. It looked like the spool player, but there was only one of the tiny, gold-colored cylinders. The other seventeen compartments were empty. "A copy, sir?"

"That's right. Maybe he can tell us how close the reproduction is."

And what about the rest of the spools? But Vancleve supposed the colonel would let him know about those if and when it suited his purpose. "Do you want him to have them today, sir? Right away?"

"No. Tomorrow, your regular visit. That'll be soon enough. But remember. We are running out of time."

He was playing the spool for himself when his office door opened and Ramachandra stuck his unruly head through, quite contrary to procedure, which required visitors to knock. But that was Ramachandra. "Ah," he exclaimed brightly, "I thought I recognized the Proxima Centauri Top Fourhundred!"

Sometimes Vancleve was dismayed at the ease with which he'd adapted to the military environment, moving from the primate ethology lab to this secret, secure facility. Ramachandra, on the other hand, would never adapt. He was a dark-skinned Puck with tangled, graying elflocks, and his rumpled UNEarth blues showed no rank insignia. They didn't even seem to be part of a uniform, worn as they were with water-buffalo leather sandals and a long embroidered vest that reached to his knees.

But he was senior to Vancleve, chief of the translation team, and definitely authorized for access to the spool player. He pulled up a chair to the desk, dropped himself into it, and settled to listen with eager enthusiasm. "Listen to that! Battling ragas—a dozen of them all at once. Just imagine if I could conduct a performance of this, what do you suppose the critics would say? 'Very avant-guard stuff. A new surrealism.' The idiots."

"You think it's just music, then, on the spools?" Vancleve asked him. "No information?"

There were several conflicting theories.

There's a code, we just haven't broken it yet.

Suppose they're recorded in another language? Why should we suppose they only have one?

Ramachandra shrugged. "Computer analysis shows less than a two percent correlation to his speech. And those sounds on the spool, those aren't voices—not even like his voice."

"So they're instruments of some kind? Musical instruments?"

"They could be anything, of course, but what's most probable? To me, it sounds like music."

He leaned forward, stabbed his finger at the player. "Hear that? It could almost be an oboe."

"Have you listened to all the spools?" Vancleve asked him.

"Actually listened to them? All eighteen spools? No, that'd be almost a thousand hours. I have them all digitized on the computer. That's what music really is, you know. Mathematics in sound."

He leaned back, crossed his legs in the chair. "So tell me how you came here, Vancleve."

Puzzled, "Someone saw a paper I'd done on nonverbal communication in primates. One day, there were two armed officers at my door. They showed me a copy of the article, ask if I'm the author. Then they offered me a proposal. I'd never seen anything like it—a security clearance? A military commission? But then I realized what must have happened, what they really wanted, and I knew I'd never have another chance like this again. I had to do it."

"Yes, it was like that with me, too," Ramachandra admitted. "I couldn't let the opportunity go, to work with an alien intelligence. You know, when I was a boy, I would see the transmissions coming back from space, the pictures of the Cloud sent by the probes. Did you know they sent out recordings on some of those early probes—sound recordings? Complete with music and voices and even photographs, too—all encoded in sound frequencies!

"I think it was then I got the notion that somehow music could be the basis for a means of universal communication. When they finally came to me and offered me the chance, how could I turn it down? Even if it meant I had to wear one of their uniforms." He grinned, knowing his contribution was too valuable for the authorities to enforce their uniform regulations in his case.

"It was Bach, wasn't it?" Vancleve asked thoughtfully. "The music they sent out into space—wasn't it Bach?"

"Ah, yes. Bach, Beethoven, folk songs. Only the difference is—we sent them the key to decode it, too. Not like this." He snorted at the spool player and uncurled his legs. "So, what are you going to do with it now?"

"Give it to him. Cho's orders."

"Ah." Ramachandra's face went sober. "I hope he enjoys his music, then."

When he was alone again, Vancleve switched off the player, sat for a long moment staring at the spool and the seventeen empty compartments in the case. Then he cued the computer, and the well-known, thin tones of a harpsichord came over the speakers: Bach. The Three-Part Inventions. He slumped in his chair with his eyes closed, losing himself in the measured beat and intricate, interwoven phrases. He could only imagine what it would be like, after five years locked up alone in an alien prison cell, to be able to hear something familiar, something from home, no matter what.

Five years.

Early the next day, getting coffee in the staff room, he turned to see Billings watching him. "I hear you're playing Good Cop for the colonel again?"

Annoyed, "Someone has to keep making an effort to communicate. Or would you rather go back to the way things were?"

God, how much more of this?

He has to crack at some point. He'll talk.

Would you?

She frowned. "You know I wouldn't. But that's not the point. You empathize. You think the alien trusts you."

His face heated slightly. The rest of the team called Billings the Skeptic. She took nothing on trust, ever.

"You think it affects my judgment?"

She shook her head, but it meant *yes*. "Just remember, without trust, there can be no betrayal. And it works both ways."

Her remarks rankled, but as always, they couldn't be dismissed. He recalled them later at the final checkpoint, when he offered Sergeant Kovic the case for inspection, along with the authorization from Colonel Cho. The sergeant trusted no one. But after Kovic had cleared it, his eyebrows raised slightly, and he asked, "What is this thing, Captain?"

"They call it a spool player. It plays music—we think."

"For *him?*" Kovic shook his head, which was as much reaction has Vancleve had ever seen from him. But four years ago he never would have asked the question.

The alien saw Vancleve come into the cell, saw what he was carrying. *"What . . ."* he asked in alien sounds incomprehensible to Vancleve but interpreted by the computer.

Vancleve knelt, offered the case. Ric moved slowly to open it, every movement and gesture registering confusion and disbelief. *"This . . . this . . . is mine, ours?"*

"It's a copy. A reproduction? Do you understand? Play it, turn it on." When Ric hesitated, he dropped the spool into the player himself.

At the first complex jumble of sound, large triangular eyes widened. The alien leaned forward, and the crest of thin, stiff hairs along the ridge of his scalp rose: auditory receptors.

What was he hearing on that disc?

"Yours, Zhrrrch? This is yours? Is this what was on the original spools? Is it the same?"

But the alien made no response, only leaned closer to the case player, as if Vancleve had never spoken, as if there were nothing else with him in the cell.

There was a monitor in Vancleve's office, and he switched it on as soon as he came back. The alien was still crouched over the spool player, eyes irised wide-open, body rocking back and forth. Vancleve watched for a few moments. There was something strangely familiar about the swaying figure. It reminded him of—what? Old men wrapped in shawls, at prayer? Was there something religious about the spools?

Since his specialty was the alien's body language, he rarely made use of the monitor's audio, but he flipped it on now, and the office again heard the complex, enigmatic alien song. What did the music mean to the alien, other than a break in his otherwise bleak and solitary existence? He did obviously recognize what the spool was playing. Whatever it was, whatever it meant.

Ramachandra thought it might only be music, but maybe he assumed too much. Billings wanted to assume nothing, but that was impossible.

Colonel Cho—wanted results.

Was the colonel using him? Using whatever trust there might be between him and the alien? Vancleve knew he was.

Any means necessary.

The next day, passing him through the checkpoint, Kovic didn't depart from procedure by as much as a single word.

Vancleve had a different case with him today. The monitor showed Ric still listening raptly to the single spool he'd brought him yesterday, but the alien looked up quickly, blinking his eyes, as soon as the door opened.

"Hello, Zhrrrch. I see you've been listening to the spool player. I hope the reproduction was good?"

His speech patterns were different, too much aware of Colonel Cho monitoring the session. He supposed it didn't make a real difference, not with the computer translating, but he tried again, "It is yours? It is sound like yours? Can you understand it?"

Slowly, Ric answered, *"Not the same. Not exactly the same. Almost."*

Vancleve took a breath. "The spools we copied this from, there were eighteen of them. That is the copy of one." He opened the case to display the rest. "Here are the others."

Ric leaned forward, drawn by the sight of them like a plant to the sunlight.

Until Vancleve said, "We would like to know what the spools say."

The alien blinked. *"They say nothing."*

Always the same answer, always the same, no matter what they tried. They could establish communication, they could force the alien to speak, but never to reveal anything they wanted to know.

"Why did your ships come so close to our space?

"Why did they fire?

"Why won't you tell us anything?"

"I know nothing."

He could be telling the truth. Maybe he really doesn't know.

He could be lying.

What if he is lying? How could we ever tell? How could we ever know, before it was too late?

Why shouldn't he lie? Wouldn't you lie, if you were in his place?

"I know nothing."

This time, Vancleve pressed for an answer. "Nothing? What have you been listening to all this time, then, if the spools say nothing?"

The alien blinked again, in (probable) confusion. *"Nothing—no words, no . . . information, data. Only tone, sound."*

Had Ramachandra been right about the spools? Vancleve wondered. "You mean, music? Songs?"

The computer digested the terms, output a string of alien sounds to which Ric responded, *"Yes, only music. No information."* And leaving Vancleve again to wonder: Was the translation module a medium for communicating with the alien or for fostering mutual confusion? How far could they rely on the computer?

But he had his instructions, and so he opened the spool case to show it more closely to Ric. "You'd like to have these, I think? Copies of the rest of the spools?"

Warily, the prisoner assented. Yes, he would like to have them.

"And we would like answers: Why your ship was near our system? Why you attacked? What will happen if we meet other ships of your people?"

Ric's six-fingered hands twitched, and his eyes blinked rapidly. *"I know nothing. I have no answers."*

What if he's lying?

What if he can't lie?

What if his memory is gone, what if they wiped it, like the computers?

This was as close to an answer as Ric had ever come before, but it wasn't enough, not with the fleet's departure date so near. Vancleve closed the case, hating himself. "I'm sorry to hear that. I'd like to give them to you, I really would. If they are only music, as you say they are. But some of our authorities think they have information."

"No. No information."

"What were they, then? Why were they on your ship?"

"I know . . . no reason . . ." Was the alien as desperate as he seemed? His body movements displayed intense signs of distress.

"Were they just entertainment?"

The translation module had a hard time with that one, but eventually Ric agreed, *"Yes, only entertainment, no information."*

"But my people need information. They need to know why your ship was here."

He'll talk. It's just a matter of time.

God, how long, though? How much more?

Hours later, he wearily opened the door to his own quarters. He fell into a chair and just sat for a moment in the silence, looking around at the familiar objects, the simple human things he took so much for granted.

After a while he got up, cued the computer, and poured out a tumbler of brandy as the sonorous depth of an organ filled the room: the Art of the Fugue.

If it had been five years, what would he give to hear Bach again—human music, any human sound? What questions would he answer? What secrets would he reveal?

"You're making progress, I'm pleased to see."

"I hope I am, sir." Vancleve knew at least one former member of the team who'd called Cho a "cold-blooded, sadistic bastard." Cho was undoubtedly cold, but Vancleve thought he was more of a pragmatist. He was willing enough to get results with kindness, as long as it worked. Using any means necessary.

"I hope it continues. You're aware that with this new launch deadline, Command has been pressuring for answers." The colonel paused, pressed his fingertips together. "But I won't give them bad answers. I'd rather admit to failure than pass on misleading information. If you get results, Captain, I want you to be sure of them."

How can we ever be sure he's not lying?

How can we be sure he understands?

It had become Vancleve's habit, in the week since he'd given Ric the spool player, to work with the audio function of his office monitor turned on. By now, he was getting somewhat used to the alien sounds—alien music.

It played ceaselessly. The alien spent every moment of the day and night crouched over the device, listening as if in a trance, swaying to a rhythm that Vancleve couldn't quite detect. Previously, when alone in the cell, he had lapsed into a motionless null state with his eyes closed, which the researchers considered the equivalent of sleep. If this was so, then he hadn't slept in all the time he'd possessed the player. His eyes were wide-open, his body in constant motion.

He spoke more now, when Vancleve came to the cell—the only times he turned the spool player off—and that was obviously for fear of having it taken away. But on all matters of importance, all the questions Command most urgently wanted answered, it was still the same: *"I don't know."*

"You don't seem to be making more progress," Colonel Cho remarked.

"No, sir."

Each spool ran for almost fifty hours of playing time. More than two days. The alien was now on the fourth, listening to each one straight through. Playing them constantly, listening constantly. To what?

Ramachandra: "Are you starting to like that stuff?"

"Getting used to it, I suppose." Vancleve looked at the monitor where Ric's image continued to crouch, to sway. "It's not monotonous. The tempo changes, but it doesn't seem to effect how he reacts."

It wasn't anything like a null state or a trance. The alien was very much alert and aware. Scans of his brain activity confirmed it. He was simply, intently listening.

Take the spools away from him, and how would he react? What would he say to get them back?

It was coming to that point, Vancleve knew. He wanted to convince Cho to let Ric finish the complete set of eighteen, but he wasn't sure of the colonel's answer. All he could do now was wait, and watch and listen along with the prisoner.

Of course the computer did most of his watching for him, ceaselessly, with the monitor as its eyes. Vancleve's programs instructed it to look for certain patterns of body language: the signs he'd interpreted as apprehension, confusion, distress. His original goal had been to determine a way to signal whether the alien was lying, but that had proved impossible; either everything Ric said was a lie or it was all the truth—or he'd failed to distinguish between them.

What if he doesn't even know the concept of a lie?

Why shouldn't he lie? Wouldn't you lie, if you were in his place?

How could they tell, without knowing what the truth was?

But as he reviewed the last night's records, he suddenly he noticed where the program had registered an anomaly, and he cut the audio, cued the monitored recording up onto the screen. Yes, it was clear—at this point Ric had started, looking up toward the door and exhibiting signs of uneasiness.

He supposed something had happened, a noise or a disturbance outside the cell. But no one had entered. Vancleve queried Security, but they reported no anomalies or disruptions that could coincide with the incident.

Frowning, he replayed it. Yes, something had

briefly agitated the prisoner while he was listening to the spool player. Was it something he'd heard?

This time, Vancleve cued the audio, and when he reached the moment that Ric flinched, his heart began to grow cold. He *recognized* that pattern of sound, distorted and altered as it was into an alien medium. The theme no longer had its original pattern and form, its voices were strange now.

Ramachandra would have known it, of course, but Ramachandra himself had never sat down to listen to the entire set of eighteen spools. The computer was infinitely faster and more accurate, but the piece had been altered so far that his programs had failed to identify it.

But the human ear, the human mind was more flexible. At last, Vancleve had learned the truth.

He cut off the monitor and closed his eyes. It wasn't betrayal. The alien had owed him nothing, his loyalty was properly to his own kind and their purposes, whatever they might have been.

And there could be no doubt of Vancleve's own, no matter how he might feel about the consequences.

It wasn't Sergeant Kovic on duty at this hour, it was another guard, but the procedure was just the same, and Vancleve was cleared to pass through the checkpoint in the usual way.

He opened the door to the cell. The alien looked up as if surprised to see him and slowly reached out to silence the spool player.

Vancleve remained standing as he said, "I want you to hear this the way it originally was, the way we made it, the way we sent it out." He cued the computer, and into the cell came the song from Earth, the bright voice of the trumpet in counterpoint to the theme of Bach's Second Brandenburg Concerto.

Once, a more innocent generation had sent that music out into anonymous space, along with greetings to any alien peoples their probe might encounter: see us, hear us, this is what we are.

Someone had heard it. Someone who had traveled to the margin of Earth's system and fired on a human ship—for whatever reasons.

"Yours, Vancleve? This is yours?"

"Ours."

The cell was monitored constantly. Soon Security would know what Vancleve had learned. Colonel Cho would. There was no concealing it. They knew the truth now, and they were rather sure that the alien prisoner had lied.

Slowly, he lowered himself to the floor next to Ric. While there was yet a little time, they knelt there together with Bach's intricate contrapuntal measures, still forever voyaging outward as other probes carried humanity's greeting to unknown alien worlds.

THE FLICKER MAN

Edward Bryant and Trey R. Barker

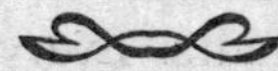

IT WAS THE KIND OF BAR WHERE ALIENS WERE KNOWN to come and drink, the town being as close as it was to the Rio Grande and all. Most strangers just appeared to wander in as chance would direct them. The place boasted no clearly discernible sign. After dark, a little neon would flicker in the windows—usually not even enough to spell out a complete brand; just some touches of bright color, that was about it.

In the daylight, not even dogs desperate for shade were inclined to go near it. But this was the hot time of the afternoon, when all sensible creatures should be sleeping.

But the woman—whose name was Ana—wasn't. Nor were the old man and the barkeep. She suddenly wanted to laugh. I *should* be sleeping, she thought. Should be sleeping for a good long time.

When she wiped her face, her hand was dry, rough with a fine, sandy dusting. No sweat, she thought wryly.

Visible waves of heat rolled through the interior of the bar, washing over the old man and the bartender. Sweat-stained napkins littered the old man's table, and when the barkeep handed him a beer, the man ran the can around his face. The barkeep sat with him and fanned himself with a torn magazine, an old copy of *Texas Monthly*.

The bar was old and as well-worn as its usual patrons, decorated with dust and grit, chipped tables and dented metal chairs. Every window along the bar's far side had a crack in it. The walls were buried behind a mob of old posters. B. B. KING LIVE! one read. MUDDY WATERS! ONE-NIGHT SHOW! blared another. Old and yellowed, held in place by cracked tape. Some of them had those ragged borders that betrayed their treatment by the kind of drinkers who killed time by carefully peeling the Lone Star stickers off the bottle in one long continuous strip.

The woman wiped her face again. Where was the sweat? Or the stains under her arms? The slick skin sliding together when her legs rubbed? The feel of ants crawling beneath her breasts? She saw the heat in the bartender's face, heard it in his grunted conversation, but she didn't feel it.

"Cain't feel what you ain't got," she said quietly to herself. And girl, she thought, you got nothin' but mad.

And the gun. She grinned. Yeah, and that.

A jukebox sat inert in the corner. The old man, stooped nearly immobile, shoved a quarter in and painfully punched up a song. A moment later, Tommy Johnson's voice came screeching from the single working speaker.

I ain't goin' down that big road by myself.
Why don't you hear me talkin', pretty mama?
Lord, ain't goin' down that big road by myself,
If I don't carry you, gonna carry somebody else.

"Gonna carry *you.*" The woman slid her hand inside her burlap bag. She squeezed her fingers around the gun butt, played idly with the trigger. Hard steel. She clicked the safety off. Wouldn't matter if she shot herself, and she didn't want the safety on when she saw him.

Sun goin' to shine in my back door someday.
And the wind goin' to change, goin' to blow my
blues away.

She shook her head. No more sun, no more wind, blues ain't going nowhere. *Nowhere.*

Out the window, the mid-afternoon sun—

A sound from the corner of the bar, like a hiccup.

—hung just at the edge of her vision. If she went outside, she would see it, and if the wind blew, she would feel it. But so what? She wasn't going to sit on the front porch tomorrow morning and let the sun warm her. Or go down to feel the breeze coming off the river. Those things were lost to her, lost like all the other little things he'd taken from her: the sun, the wind, the rain, walks in the park, delivered pizza. And the big—

A sound like a short laugh. Loud in the bar, blaring in her ears. Then a low static.

—things? She shook her head. Thinking about the big things led her to Sally and she desperately didn't want to think of Sally. Little Sally lost, little Sally gone forever.

Ana slammed her fist against the bar. The two men ignored her.

The hum grew, like someone turning up the volume on a radio station not tuned in very well. Ana glanced back into the corner and realized the sound wasn't static. It was a pained moan.

Light flickered.

The man flickered.

She saw him before he actually appeared. Like the sun's afterimage when you look quick. There was a man there, but not really there, though she could hear his howl. Ana looked up. The bartender and the old man didn't seem to hear anything of what was going on in the corner where the flickering and the howling were raising quite a ruckus.

Part of him flickered into view and then back out. Each time he came back, there was a bit more of him. An arm, a chest, a leg.

Christ, what's this? She was still uncertain enough about herself to wonder what else she might see. Was this guy like her? Even worse? Trembling, she gripped the gun tighter.

And then he was all the way there. Slumped over a corner table, breathing heavily.

She cast a quick look toward the bartender. Over the top of his glasses, he looked at her for a moment, then turned away. He still didn't see the new arrival.

Finally, a little scared, Ana stared at the guy. His color was faded. Not from being sick pale, but like a drawing the artist hadn't colored completely. The brown of his hair, the white of his skin. Even the blue of his jeans and the red of his shirt were faded.

"Something wrong?" the bartender asked. The old man snickered.

"Uh . . . no." With a curt nod, she turned back to the flickering man. But even as her hand tightened on the gun, her fear slipped away. She wasn't scared of the new guy, though maybe she should be. Maybe her signals were just screwed up. Maybe she should be terrified. Except there was nothing for her fear to grab. There were none of the petty threats she'd felt in the last three days; none of the monstrous threats that left her convinced someone was about to die brutally. All the threats that haunted living people's hearts and swam in her own head were absent from this man.

Then the flickering man winked out of existence.

And returned.

While she watched, his face faded into view again, features twisting as his hands grabbed at the table. The quiet static climbed the scale to an ear-splitting scream, though neither the barkeep nor the customer seemed to notice yet.

Finally, he raised his head. A thin line of blood leaked from a slightly askew nose. He looked at her a moment, then tried to smile. The smile faded when he saw Ana staring at him. "You can see me?"

She nodded.

"Hmmm, that's something new. Well, if you can see me, I guess I made it."

"If this is where you want to be, you made it, for damn sure." She licked her lips. "Goddamned if I don't need a beer or three. Hey, I need a—" She turned to the man. "You wanna beer? Two beers," she called to the bartender. No response. The fury kicked in. *"Now!"*

The bartender grumbled as he brought them. "Drinking alone?" He shook his head, then set the bottles down without napkins and left as soon as she paid.

Ana shoved a beer toward the man across the table and slammed back a huge swallow of her own. The man stared at the bottle for a moment, then drank. He frowned as he swallowed. "I've had better," he said.

"Ain't we all?"

He took another large gulp. "Home brew, New York speakeasy, nineteen twenty-three. *That* was good."

Ana stared at him, puzzled. He was a few years older than she, but damn sure not old enough to guzzle beer in some piss-hole seventy years ago. Staring at him through the bottom of the clear bottle, she finished her beer.

He drained his own bottle and pushed it away. His eyes, hard as steel now, not the faded things she'd seen earlier, focused on her. He stared until she felt the flush invade her cheeks. She looked around the bar, avoiding his gaze. When she could stand it no longer, Ana glared at him. "What the hell're you staring at?"

"You're not like them." He nodded toward the bartender and the old man.

It wasn't a question, but simple fact. She was nothing like the two men and he knew it. She shrugged. It made them even because he wasn't anything like the other two men, and she was beginning to understand he wasn't anything like her, either.

"No, I ain't like them," she said. "And neither're you."

He extended a hand. "I am called Param." He shrugged. "Perhaps we are two of a kind."

At the front of the bar, the old man stood and shuffled slowly back toward the jukebox. He eyed Ana the entire way. At the jukebox, he shoved in another quarter, punched more numbers, then scooted back to the front table.

She ignored Param's offered hand and shook her head. "I'm Ana and we ain't two of a kind 'cause you ain't nothing like me." She knew she was confirming it to herself.

His right eyebrow raised. "Oh? And what are you?"

A low, mournful E minor chord on a slightly out of tune guitar slipped hesitantly from the jukebox. A heavy voice followed.

I went down to the St. James Infirmary.
I saw my baby there.
Stretched out on a long white table.
So sweet, so cold, so fair.

She nodded. "That's me. The dead part, anyway."

"Yes," Param said quietly, as though considering the thought for the first time. "Yes, indeed, that is you, isn't it?"

"Yeah. I think I'm a ghost, but I really ain't got no idea." A frustrated sigh slipped between her lips. Almost like a final breath.

The door burst open, spilling a big, loud, laughing man into the bar. Both Ana and the flicker man—as she now thought of him—jumped. She whirled and stared at the new arrival. "That's the asshole who did it," she said, ripping the pistol from the burlap bag.

"Hey!" the big man called, closing the door with a bang and sitting himself down at the front table next to the old man. "There he is, the best barkeep in the world."

The bartender shook his head. "No free booze this time, Charley."

"Shit, no, I got bread, courtesy of a brand-new customer. A round for everybody."

A new customer. Ana stiffened, gripped the pistol so tight her fingers ached.

The old man mumbled a tired cheer. The barkeep shook his head. "Real impressive, Charley. Only three people in here, you asshole."

Charley grinned and surveyed the rest of the dimly lit bar. When he saw Ana, his eyes went wide. "What the hell?" His expression froze in shock.

Ana stood and leveled the Beretta smoothly, just like Charley had shown her in a different time. Ease back the hammer, she thought. Line your sight, squeeze the trigger gently.

"Ana?" Param called, his voice bordering on panic. "What are you doing?"

She ignored Param, her own eyes hard as she stepped toward her father. "Surprised? Thought you'd taken care of it all, didn't you?"

"Christ," the bartender muttered. "Come on, Ana, what's going on?"

Charley seemed to wrench his composure back forcibly. He held his arms out wide, palms up. "Hey, look, little girl, you're pretty lively for a corpse. Guess maybe I wasn't as rough on you as I thought. You sure you wanna wave that thing around so casual like?"

"Yeah, pretty sure," Ana said grimly. She gave her father a smile that was all teeth. "And yes, I *am* pretty lively for a corpse." She moved into the light and everyone stared at her midsection, where she held the Beretta.

"Oh shit, Charley," the barkeep said. "Do something about this. I don't need to spend the day cleaning your guts off my wall."

"He ain't got nothing to say over this. And I'm sorry it had to happen here." She shrugged. "Just the way things work out, I guess."

"Ana," Param said quietly. He moved near her. "This isn't right. Put that weapon down."

Ana laughed. "Ain't right? Ain't fucking *right?*" She lunged forward, shoving the Beretta smack into Charley's face. The blued steel barrel clicked against his teeth. Charley yelped and recoiled. "What *you* did was right? Selling me outta the back of your truck? Killing me 'cause I didn't want it no more?"

"Obviously I didn't kill you *too* dead," Charley muttered.

"Shut up!" Ana screamed. "Not another fucking word or I'll end it here and now." The men watched as, with her free hand, she unconsciously tucked something slick and leathery, something that had come loose, back into the hole in her belly.

"You need a sawbones," said Charley. A quick look passed over his face. Slowly, he lowered his hands. "Sounds like you got something you wanna talk over, little girl."

"I need a priest, Daddy. Call me little girl again and the barkeep'll be cleaning this bar all night."

Charley, grinning, shook his head. "I don't think so."

"Ana, please," Param said. A sheen of sweat danced across his brow. "What's done is done. Can it change anything to kill him?"

"Stay out of this." Ana didn't turn her face away from Charley. "It'd change one thing, maybe. Right, Charley?"

Charley glanced at the old man and the barkeep. They stood near the far wall, eyes intent on Ana, definitely not eager to play heroes or get in the line of fire. "I . . . I don't know what you're talking about," he said.

Ana thumbed the hammer back. "Bullshit."

"Come on, now, Ana," Charley whispered. "Sally needs you."

She wanted to cry. As clear as the morning run of trucks along the highway, Ana heard Charley's breath rumbling hoarsely. He's scared, Ana thought.

Yes, and you've done it to him.

The voiceless whisper was soft, though it pounded in her head like a sledgehammer. She jerked her gaze toward Param. He nodded slightly. *You can't kill him, Ana, waste of flesh though he may be. It's just not ri—*

The whisper stopped suddenly, replaced by a vocalized shout. "Charley, no, don't—"

Ana turned just as Charley lunged at her. His laugh, maddened by fear, rang through the old bar. Ana jerked the trigger and the first shot went wild, shattering a light fixture before leaving a hole in the ceiling. Plaster dust showered down. The second shot nicked Charley's arm and slammed between the eyes of a dusty mounted javelina head hanging crooked on the wall.

Howling, Charley grabbed his arm. Blood leaked between his fingers. Behind him, the barkeep and the old man darted out the door. The trophy javelina bounced to the plank floor and rolled. Ana squinted, and squeezed the trigger five times.

Five bullets exploded from the gun and slammed into a soft blue glow hovering a few inches in front of Charley. He fell back across a table, mouth open in terror though Ana heard nothing but the gun's bark. When she released the trigger and the shooting stopped, she stared at Charley. The blue light had wrapped itself around him. His scream was weak, as though he were standing clear across town.

Furious, she turned to Param. "You did this!" She kicked at Charley. Her foot slipped into the blue light as though it were pudding, the sharp motion abruptly stalled. She jerked it free. "Get him out!"

"I'm sorry, Ana, I can't."

"Bullshit!"

"I can't let you kill him."

She turned back to Charley, his mouth still open and eyes tightly closed, and emptied the clip. Charley jumped at each report, but Ana never saw the blood she so desperately wanted to see.

A distant siren began to swell. Ana stared at Charley, then glanced at Param. Anger overwhelmed her. She'd been so close and yet this . . . *thing* had stopped her, had refused her the satisfaction she needed.

"Listen, Ana," the flicker man said. "You're dead. Killing this man will do nothing. Why end another life simply because he ended yours? Why let yourself wallow in shallow revenge?"

Ana shook her head as though dealing with a painfully slow child. "You don't understand. It's not just me, there's another—"

In a spray of gravel and noise, the sheriff's car skidded to a stop in the parking lot.

"In spite of your death, you have still have a physicality, and if they clap you in jail, I doubt you will get out."

Ana shrugged. "I don't know. I got no idea what I can and can't do. I only been dead three days." She leaned toward the blue glow enfolding Charley and spat. The saliva slowed, stopped, fell.

"Lazarus woman," Param said, gently touching her shoulder. "Come," he said decisively. He guided her through the sudden blackness.

The dark was endless, like staring into a bottomless lake. Could you lose yourself in it? Could you lose yourself in a sense of complete comfort? In the complete relaxation?

Hell no, Ana thought she whispered.

Could you go mad?

Unable to stop it now, she could see the madness coming, hidden inside the blackness that had seduced her with its massaging touch. She would be conscious of it even as it happened. And when she was helpless, she would know it but wouldn't care.

Because this blackness was all she wanted. Peace. Quiet. Comfort. No screaming daddies you couldn't fight, no crying daughters you couldn't help. There might not be a pleasant rain or gentle breeze in this place, but there was no sticky slime left on her belly or blood staining her thighs.

No, none of that, Param said. Except he didn't speak.

With no head to turn, no eyes with which to see, Ana looked around. She didn't see Param's face, but she knew he was near, floating in the blackness where he'd brought her. She felt the steady rhythm of his heartbeat, the cool warmth of his breath.

What the hell is this place? Ana thought Param shrugged, though she saw nothing.

Nowhere, really. Or everywhere, depending on how you look at it.

That ain't no answer. Ana sighed. Except there was no sound, only silence. *You should'a let me kill him. He's a shit.*

Perhaps he is. I don't know. But I couldn't let you take his life.

Oh, yeah, it ain't right. Ain't that what you said?

For a long time, maybe forever, maybe only a split second, Param said nothing. The silence around them was complete, like when she first woke up after

Charley shot her. Silence penetrated as thoroughly as any of Charley's friends. Or his "customers."

You won't go mad here, Ana. After all, how can the dead be mad?

If I'm dead, what the hell am I doing here? She wanted desperately to cry, or scream or pound a fist through a cheap wall. Anything to relieve the pressure, the anxiety.

Tell me about Sally.

She said nothing, but thoughts of the girl roared through her head. Little Sally lost. Left with no mother. Left with a man who sold his own daughter for booze money. Left with a man who'd sell his granddaughter eventually, if he hadn't already. Left with a man she would eventually die for, one way or another.

Your name is Anastasia.

Ana snorted. *Yeah, what of it?*

Do you know what it means?

Who gives a shit? When can I go home? I got some business to finish.

It means, Param said, as though he hadn't heard, *resurrected.*

Who gives a shit?

Her tears came suddenly, unexpectedly, sheeting like summer rain. Face or not, she could feel warm tears slipping down her cheeks, dropping off the edge of her sharp chin. At least this darkness could let her cry.

You got a little girl's name for dead?

No.

The name's Sally, that's the name for dead.

I don't think so. I think she's alive, smiling and

laughing and singing songs. Sally is a form of Sarah. It means princess.

You don't know Charley. She ain't doin' no smiling or laughing or singing with him. *I can guarantee it.*

I don't understand.

Why'd you bring me here? I could have saved Sally.

Most every night, when Ana was a little girl, her father had come home drunk. Sometimes he passed out on the couch, sometimes he pounded Mama before passing out. Sometimes he sat in his chair and asked Mama questions that mostly had no answers. Ana had always been able to feel her mother's confusion. It had been thick like morning fog or summer heat. Now, she felt Param's confusion the same way.

Saved her? I don't understand. She's not dead.

One shot, between his eyes, right in his gut or his chest, it don't matter. Ana laughed loud. If it had been a real sound, it would have boomed through the dark.

Maybe blow his balls off. Poetic justice.

Why?

'Cause he's got Sally now. And all Sally had was me, bad as that was, but now she ain't got shit. Nothing but that asshole Charley.

Your father.

She snorted.

Once't, maybe, but not for a long time now. Bastard sold me outta his truck. Sat in the cab listening to music while men grunted and sweated over me in the camper.

Again the silence, but now Ana found she could breathe, that it didn't press against her as badly.

Gettin' used to it? Gettin' used to the peace and quiet? Maybe forgettin' what Charley sounds like when he's bargaining with a guy over a blow job from his kid? *His* princess?

Finally, Param spoke again. He had come near her, perhaps just beyond the tips of her fingers.

So many worlds, so many universes. More than most people can imagine.

Ana heard what could have been a quiet laugh. Or a broken sigh.

So many places with so many problems. Only a few worlds I would call perfect. Not really *perfect, but close enough. I keep looking, though, trying to find the one I need.*

What are you doing here? Ana asked tiredly.

Traveling, like you.

I ain't traveling nowhere.

Aren't you? You've left life behind and—

Fucker stole it.

Perhaps, but you've left it behind and now you're looking for something new.

I'm just tired, Param. Damn tired. I don't want to look for a new nothing. I just want to keep Sally safe and go to sleep. Why can't I do that?

I don't know. I've been here before, this place . . . this world of yours. New York City, Madrid, Constantinople, Rome under the triumvirate, the Sumerian city of Ur.

Ain't my world. Be a helluva lot different if it were.

I've visited before, always by myself. I've never seen one quite like you.

I've seen a few, wandering around, crying and pissing. Moaning about shit.

You miss your daughter, don't you?

Ain't you the genius.

You talked to the bartender, though. And to Charley. You're not completely alone, are you? They can see you, they can talk to you. I don't have that ability.

He was silent for a while. *I think I know. They hear you and see you because you have so strong a need to be heard and seen. Your passion is to save your daughter. Even death can't stop you.*

Then, almost forlornly, *No one's ever felt that passion for me.*

A terrible thought occurred to her. She grappled with it silently at first, then lashed out. *You brought me here because you're fucking* lonely?

Anger welled up. She felt her hands clenching to fists, though she couldn't see them. She felt her heart speed up, pounding in her chest. Because he was lonely? Damn him.

I could have saved my daughter and now she's probably dead because you needed somebody to talk to? Because I can hear you? *Are you crazy?*

I just didn't realize. I'm sorry. I didn't know about Sally. I knew you couldn't kill Charley because it was wrong.

Says who? 'Cause they don't kill in your perfect worlds?

He laughed. *Not my worlds. I've no worlds of my own anymore, but in the best worlds I've seen, the ones I've gone back to, there is no killing.*

Well, there's killing here, and now that you've fucked things up, Sally's part of that killing. She's dead.

No. I keep telling you, she's not dead. She still lives.

Ana bit down on her anger.

Then take me back. Let me help her. Damn it, she's my daughter.

You'll stop your father by killing him.

Yes! She wanted to shout, to scream. *Yes yes yes! How else? Damn it, you freak, let me go home.*

I'm sorry, Ana. I thought you were lonely. I thought I could give you friendship.

I don't have time for lonely. I want my daughter.

Ana frowned. Want her? Sure, she did, but she figured there was no way that was going to happen. All Ana could do was try to save her daughter and hope for the best. And now, that might not even be possible. Who the hell *knew* what the rules of death were?

She felt Param close to her. His breath on her neck, a hand light on her shoulder.

I am sorry, Ana.

The black faded—

—and became night, outside the bar. Of the four streetlights in the parking lot, only one worked. It cast a weak piss-yellow glow on the far side of the lot, leaving Charley's camper truck shrouded in near complete dark.

"Param." Ana looked around, waiting for him to appear. Bastard would have to be there, to stop her from killing Charley. The lot remained empty. Param had not come back with her.

Ana took a deep breath and headed for the truck. A scratchy old blues number came from the cab. Loud enough, Ana thought with a grim smile, to wake the dead.

The sky is crying, look at the tears roll
down the street.
The sky is crying, look at the tears roll
down the street.
I been looking for my baby,
And I wonder where can she be?

Walking slowly, clenching and letting go her fists, Ana shuddered. Most likely, her baby was in that truck. Most likely, her baby was getting pawed by some drunk. Most likely her baby was calling for Mama. While Charley sat and listened to the music, and dreamed of his next big score.

Her ragged nails bit into the center of her palms. She half-expected to feel warm blood dance down her hands. There was none, just as there was no blood coming from the huge hole Charley had blown in her gut. Or the broken nose Charley had smashed with the gun butt. And certainly none from all the wounds he'd given her in the past, the bruises, the torn places inside where you couldn't see, the scars from the cigarette burns.

"Too late t' worry about that," she whispered, patting the pistol tucked in her waistband. "Just save your baby."

She heard the sound of shuffling feet from the other side of the camper shell, a slightly out of tune hum, the lyric screwed up. Ana knew the shuffle, knew the voice that sounded always like its owner had a head cold. She knew the smell of his sweat and the way he liked to talk like a baby when he screwed. She knew how he liked to see blood.

"Bullshit," she whispered, jerking the Beretta

from her pants waist. She felt a stab of panic. Had she emptied the clip? Didn't matter now. "Ain't bleeding my girl."

She aimed the pistol in the direction of the humming, though she couldn't see the man. A second later, his dark face emerged into the dim light. It was one of the prick bastards Charley called his customers. Ana grinned at the sudden fear that sculpted his features.

"Whoa now, Ana," he said. "What the fuck is this?"

She spoke slowly. "Get outta here or I'll blast you to fucking Kingdom Come."

"Whassa' matter," he asked, his voice slipping into baby-talk. "Din' you like how your Pa treated you? Din' he give you—"

"Shut up!" She shoved the gun into his face and jerked back the hammer.

"Fine, fine, crazy bitch." He turned and disappeared into the night.

The cab door clattered and screeched open.

"What the hell is—" Charley stopped short as he exited the cab. "Jesus Christ."

Ana jerked the gun around and stuck it in his face. The shaking in her hands made it seem as though she were aiming for both his eyes, the barrel moving between them.

"Get her out."

"Or what? You'll shoot me?" He grinned and did a little dance step. "I don't think so. You done tried that, remember? You tried and you couldn't do it." He laughed.

When she pulled the trigger, the gun only clicked.

The hand that smashed against her head was a

blur, a stain of solid flesh in the dim light. She fell violently to the ground though there was no pain. When she looked up, a boot flashed out, knocking the gun from her hand. Charley's foot swung back again, landing once with a soft squashy sound in her gut and once against her head.

"You didn't want ol' Slim gettin' inta Sally's pants? Well, then, I guess I'll just have to do it myself. It's a father's job." He pulled some keys from his pocket and unlocked the camper door, unzipping his dirty jeans with his free hand. As soon as the door popped open, Sally exploded from the inside, screaming and pounding at Charley's face.

They tumbled to the ground, angry screams mixed with pained howls. Sally slammed her knee repeatedly into Charley's crotch and scratched at his face with her stubby fingernails.

"Baby?" Ana said, surprised by Sally's fierce anger. Her daughter was all of nine.

As she landed a punch to Charley's gut, Sally looked toward Ana. Her eyes opened wide in surprise. Her blow fell soft. "Mama?"

In that split second, Charley slammed his meaty fist into Sally's chin. The girl's head snapped to the side, banging against the truck. A howl gurgled and died in Sally's throat. He landed one more blow before Ana got to him.

"Get off me, bitch," Charley yelled.

Ana shoved herself against him. A weak, off-balance punch landed against her temple. She raised a protective hand but Charley hit low. Reeling, she staggered away, wondering suddenly if Charley could beat to death a woman he'd already killed.

"Come on back," Charley threatened. "Get another one, I'll give it to you all night!"

When Ana looked up, Charley had pulled Sally to her feet and had her head cupped in his hand. He leaned her back slightly and then shoved her forward, toward the truck's tailgate. "Here's a little present for your bitch kid."

"No!"

Ana surged forward, knowing she was too far away. She got there just as he smashed Sally's head into the tailgate, just as blood sprayed the truck, just as Sally died.

"Sally!"

When she reached him, Charley raked a forearm across Ana's face. Ana stumbled backward as a shaft of intense blue light slipped sideways through the night. It moved across the truck and past Sally, then sliced through Charley. It was a carving knife honed of light.

His scream was short and Ana felt cheated. She wanted to hear it long and loud, like the wail of a triumphant guitar. She wanted to hear Charley's scream over and over and remember it forever. She wanted to play it like an old 45 record, throwing it on the turntable whenever she wanted so she could always listen to it.

"Ahhhh . . . damn . . ." Drool dribbled down Charley's chin as he slumped to the ground. He released Sally and she fell in a heap. A second later, Charley collapsed over her.

The hum charged the air like an electrical storm. Ana knelt at her daughter's side and pushed Charley off her. She looked around the parking lot. Near the center of the deserted concrete, the dark was deeper than the night.

"Param," Ana said, cradling her daughter. "Please . . . help her."

Quicker than in the bar, Param flickered into view. A shapeless gray appeared, slipping into a gray shadow and then Param. His color was faded, his face sallow and pinched, his eyes empty. He stared at Charley until Ana spoke.

"Help her, Param. I know you can."

He shook his head. "I can't, Ana. She's dead."

"No, she can't be . . . I saved her . . . I tried to save her . . . I tried—"

"Ana, let her go. She's dead."

"So am I!" Ana yelled. "But *I'm* here." She leaned over Sally, kissing the girl's bloody face. She rocked gently. "Oh, God. I love you, Sally."

"Ana, she didn't want to live as fiercely as you did. She didn't have the same passion to come back."

She glared at him. "I could have saved her, you fuck! I could have saved her!" Ana set Sally's body down and lunged at Param.

He stood still and let Ana collide with him. They fell to the pavement, Ana's fists pummelling Param's face and chest.

"She's dead 'cause of you!" Ana screamed.

Param nodded, not bothering to shield his face. "I know. I know. I'm sorry."

How long can I go, Ana wondered. My hands won't get bloody. I won't get tired. Can I beat him forever? Can I kill him? She wanted to kill him. She wanted him as dead as Charley and Sally. She wanted him to suffer and die slowly.

"I won't die, Ana." Param finally grabbed her fists and held them away from his face. "Beat me forever and I won't die, I tried to tell you that."

Ana fell away from Param, crying even though no tears came. Sally was dead and though it was his fault, at the same time, it *wasn't* his fault. Charley would have killed her eventually, just as he had done with Ana. And until then, Sally would have been endlessly raped, just as Ana had been. "When I was alive, I protected her," Ana said, sliding her arm back under Sally's body. "I couldn't do that and be dead. I couldn't do anything for her."

"Except kill Charley."

Ana nodded and kissed Sally's face a final time. Then she stood. "Why'd you do it?"

Param spoke quietly. "For the same reason you wanted to." He shrugged. "I'm sorry, Ana. You told me but I didn't understand, not in time."

The first shriek of a siren rose in the distance.

"I guess somebody heard the fight," Ana said.

"I am sorry, Ana."

Ana nodded. "Ain't nothin' to be done now, she's dead. At least she won't have to go through what I did. Maybe it's better, I don't know."

Param nodded and began walking away.

Ana bit back another bout of crying. Sally wasn't better off dead, she was just dead and she wasn't going to wake up like Ana had. There was nothing left now. She glanced at her daughter, then at Charley, then at Param's back. "Where you goin'?" she asked quietly.

He stopped. "This isn't the place I thought it was. It's time to go somewhere else."

"You runnin' away?"

Param shook his head. "Maybe. I always thought I was just looking. I'm a searcher."

Ana cocked her head curiously. "My ma used to talk about that wonderin' Jew guy. You him?"

"No, Ana." Param actually smiled. "I think you mean *wandering*."

"How about that flying Dutchman, you know, the sailor?"

"I'm an explorer. I look for worlds."

Ana hesitated. "Um . . . how 'bout showin' me some of those worlds."

Param said nothing.

"Why not? I ain't got nothing left here. Only person I loved is dead and I'm still here. I didn't suddenly go to Heaven or anywhere. I guess maybe I'm here to stay."

Param was quiet for a moment. "Perhaps there is a reason."

"Like?"

The siren was closer, only a few blocks away now. Param stared toward the sound, took a deep breath, and nodded. "We will figure it out later."

Ana realized she was smiling. Not much of a smile, but it was a start. "Knock yourself out," she said.

A moment later, they inhabited the blackness again, but this time a darkness studded with countless pinpricks of brilliant white light.

The dots of light flickered.

Then burned steady and true.

GUESSING AT THE UNKNOWN

Cindie Geddes

I WAS TEN WHEN MY FATHER WALKED OUT. I REMEMBER because that was the same summer the aliens came. Not that I wouldn't have remembered anyway. Things like that tend to retain their importance over the years.

Unlike the aliens.

It's hard now, fourteen years later, to remember how excited we all were when the news was released. The near-euphoria, the relief, the almost religious fervor with which the country welcomed the strangers lit the days with a sense of abandon and something I only later learned to identify as desperation. Our own reaction took us all a little by surprise. Even we children were confused by the sudden lifting of restrictions, by the playfulness of our parents, the whimsy of our teachers.

My mother, though her life had so recently been

thrown into a shambles, was humming and smiling as she watched the news while preparing our dinner. "Now this is something," she told me as the steam from the mac and cheese sent her hair into tight curls around her face. "This will change everything."

I grinned and nodded, just happy to see a smile light her eyes once again. Since my father's abrupt departure a month and a half earlier (and how long could it possibly take to get a pack of cigarettes anyway?) her smiles had been wide, toothy monstrosities that only left me cold. But now that the aliens had come, eight short hairless grinning creatures, her eyes were bright and her words musical with a depth of tone that I had thought lost.

"Intelligent life," she said as she filled my plate with my favorite cheesy food. "Imagine how surprised Congress must be. It's been a long time since Washington's seen any."

I laughed along with her though I wasn't sure what she meant. It felt good. *We* felt good. All thanks to the aliens.

That night she let me stay up late and watch the news with her. The aliens shaking hands (if you could call their fused, flipperlike appendages hands) with the president. Aliens accompanied by blue-suited Secret Service men as they explored a Haight-Ashbury clothing store in San Francisco, trying on hats over their tiny, bald heads, and wearing bell bottoms that were as wide as they were, and army boots wiggling with every step of their small, fused feet. In hindsight, they didn't look any more ridiculous than their hippy counterparts, but we thought they were a riot back then.

"Aliens in San Francisco," Mom smiled. "Carl would love this." She fiddled with the beaded tassels on her leather vest and I heard it in her voice. It only took a second for her face to fall and then the fake smile to reappear. "Your daddy loves science fiction." She laughed too loudly. "Although I guess this is science fact."

I tried to bring the music back to her voice, to chase away the stressed, high pitch of her lies—subtle lies to reassure me he was coming back. "Their heads are weird," I said, my own voice rising in its attempt at diversion.

"Honey, lots of people are bald," she laughed and the laugh was a little looser.

"Not like that," I said as I mimicked the completely hairless aliens in berets and floppy leather hats, admiring themselves and each other in the mirrors.

In a flash, she went to her room and came back with a handful of hats that we tried on ourselves in the glow of the evening news, aping around the room, copying the aliens' slow, awkward movements, laughing at ourselves and each other. And I knew my father was, for the moment, forgotten.

The aliens were given U.S. citizenship before I started school that same year they arrived. We wanted the aliens all to ourselves and citizenship seemed the best way to accomplish the goal. It worked. The aliens showed no interest in travel at all. For stellar explorers, they were remarkable homebodies. And we understood. America had everything anyone could want. It made us proud.

After the citizenship, began the research. "I'm surprised it took them this long," my mom said as we heard the news on the car radio as she picked me up from school. "Didn't want to force them, I guess."

"They couldn't do that, could they?" I asked.

"Honey, in this country, the government can do anything they want."

"But I thought—"

"Anything they want. It's not right, but it's the truth."

We listened to the radio, through the news report, past an amazingly irritating disco-laden advertisement for Ditto Jeans, to the beginning of a song my mom and dad used to dance to. Simon and Garfunkel. "Bridge Over Troubled Water." I knew every word to every song on that album. We used to sing "Cecilia" at the top of our lungs on camping trips. If it rained, we sang "The Boxer," stumbling over the words until someone started to giggle. But "Bridge Over Troubled Water" was always for dancing. I still remember watching my parents dancing on the back lawn, wine glasses at their feet, roach in the ashtray, mellow cords drifting up to the stars on the backbeat of promises.

I watched the look on her face as she reached out slowly to the volume knob, hesitated, and switched it off with authority. She looked older than I'd ever seen her. Her straight blond hair was limply pulled into a ponytail; wrinkles marred her perfect features, deepening as she scowled. "I never liked them," she said quietly.

I let her have her silence. And her lies.

When we got home, she turned her attention to the

news and immersed herself in the stories of the aliens. They never ceased to amaze her.

Everyone was fascinated by the aliens. And the aliens loved the attention. News shows gave us glimpses of the posh housing the government had set up, the fine food and even finer clothing brought in on drab green trucks. Papers reported on the testing—interviews and psych test, intelligence evaluations and physicals. Some even ran copies of the aliens' rather simplistic answers. The aliens and their test results occupied the media for months. Every picture showed a smile, every report had a kitschy quote from one of our eight friends. We thought our visitors had found their niche—perennial students.

It was summer again when the word was announced. Everyone was taken aback. How could this be? But the truth was in the scores. The aliens had flunked.

They had nothing to offer us. Not new technology, not advanced culture, not even an interesting language (we'd figured that out before the tests even began).

The aliens were stupid.

Their ship was recovered from an alien crash on their own planet and then tested by their planet's leading scientists. The alien scientists had just recently discovered the combustible engine and were no better equipped to decipher the craft's technology than were our own. With little forethought and absolutely no idea what they were doing, they had jumped in their new toy and taken it for a spin—amazingly, it flew—and ended up here.

The language was easy. The rest took longer, because we were simply not ready for the results.

Their culture was based on material wealth and personal appearance. A rudimentary system of trade was based on carved representations of one another with weighted value given to the most attractive of their species.

Government was hereditary, but in a society that valued sloth, leadership was often abdicated to those considered too homely to be of any other service.

Then there was the matter of the reproduction—spontaneous, asexual reproduction that could produce a fully grown alien in two weeks. During their first year on our planet, the eight original aliens reproduced rapidly, but that was it. Before we even had a chance to figure out how they did it, they were done.

Now there were over two hundred, and the government no longer wanted them.

It was a few weeks after my fifteenth birthday when I next heard from my dad. But by then, it wasn't a really big deal. I'd gotten used to him being gone, and had even come to like having it be just me and my mom. We were pals, more like sisters than mother and daughter, and all my friends envied me. No one else's mom was as cool as mine. Or as pretty. I stayed out as late as I wanted, though never as late as she did; I could go to any movie that interested me, could skip school whenever I liked as long as my grades didn't slip.

So I didn't much miss not having a strong male role model. I had plenty of males around, just none I considered a dad. And why not—Mom never considered any of them a husband. Then when I got the letter, I was sure I wasn't missing anything. My father was working as a garbage man in Florida, living on the streets, suicidal, and still evidently unable to kick the drugs that had plagued him for as long as I could remember. He tried to explain why he left—wrote that he was afraid of screwing up my and Mom's life. I had to respect that. Though he could've found a better way to go about it. Mostly, I just felt sorry for him. Seemed his life had gone to hell since he left, while mine and Mom's couldn't be better.

There was no return address.

Mom gave me the letter; I read it; she stuck it in a box. It should've been a big deal, a momentous occasion, something of emotional import, but it wasn't. My mind was busy worrying about other things—whether Jeff would find out I'd gone to a movie with Chris, whether Mrs. Madison would really make me start coming to class every day, whether or not NASA would ever be able to test the alien spacecraft.

After their population stopped growing, the aliens became even more popular. Despite science's professed boredom, we were still fascinated by the hairless wonders. They were everywhere—magazine covers, television sitcoms and soaps, talk shows, strip mall grand openings, political campaigns. No matter where you looked, they were there—bald heads the size of softballs, wedgelike hands in waves and grand sweeping gestures, stumpy little feet dangling off swings and diving boards, advertising everything from jeans to juicers and making the cover of every trash paper in the country with their antics. The seemingly sexless creatures dated sports legends and rock idols, movie stars and super models; they campaigned for Democrats and rallied behind Republicans, read the weather and announced pee-wee football games. Every event had to have an alien.

And to think the government was worried how our country would support them and their now-lavish tastes.

By the time I was fifteen, the aliens were celebrities. But that was all they were. And it was enough. They didn't contribute to science or medicine or education or the arts, though a few did become lawyers.

The ship, however, its origin still completely unknown, was proving useful. Five years of constant research, billions of dollars spent, and we were finally beginning to understand the alien craft. Space would be ours. Or so we hoped.

Fame doesn't last forever. And every child grows bored with even their most loved toy. As did we. Our aliens grew tiresome. And they grew older. Much older. They aged so much more quickly than we did, their medical costs were astronomical.

No insurance—the aliens had never worked.

No money—they never grasped the concept that their looks would not be enough.

No fans—when the celebrities began to avoid them, we all did.

Suddenly the politicians and the businessmen and

the advertisers no longer needed them. Neither did we. But what could we do? They were ours.

At twenty-two, I started wondering about my baby's grandpa. Cili (who still couldn't or wouldn't say Cecilia) was five and precocious and curious about everything around her. She didn't remember her grandma, who died in a car wreck a few days before my baby's second birthday. And it wasn't until she started preschool that she became curious about relations others had but she didn't. She understood that she had no aunts and uncles because I was an only child too. She understood that her father sent checks and visited every other weekend (after all, didn't everybody's). But she didn't understand grandparents. Or, more precisely, why she didn't have any.

Death was still a mystery to her, but not as much as the idea that she had a grandpa that I knew nothing about. I think it was because of my lack of knowledge she became curious. And then I became curious. My own brief marriage (we never even celebrated an anniversary) had been a simple mistake. Just wasn't meant to be. The divorce was mutual and friendly and Sean and I are still good friends. No regrets.

The comparisons to my mom's marriage were inevitable, I suppose. After all, despite the leaving part, it was what I had wanted. My memories are still filled with glimpses of their romance. Dancing, chasing one another, love notes pinned to the refrigerator, warm champagne on hot summer nights. Ten good years. I didn't even have one.

So what had happened? Ten years, for Christ's sake. That's a long time. Then one day—that's it—he's gone? Just left a wife and kid to fend for themselves (which we did quite well, thank you very much).

It's the leaving the kid part I don't understand. Threat of death would not make me leave Cili. But if I had a drug problem . . . If I couldn't take care of her . . . If my staying threatened to ruin her life . . . I don't know. Who am I to say? Time changes people. Changes the world. Nothing stays the same, so how do I know what my father's life turned into. What if he got off drugs, remarried, had a new wife and kids? Who'd want to be reminded of the past then?

And what if he was dead?

I answered Cili's questions honestly and tried to explain that we wouldn't be seeing her grandpa. She didn't understand.

"Why not?"

"Because I don't know where he is."

"Find out."

"How?" I laughed.

"The same way they're finding the aliens."

"It's not the same. The government is looking for the aliens. Not just a normal person."

"I don't think it's fair."

"Not everything is, honey."

"Everything should be."

How could I argue that? She was right. Rounding up the aliens—all 208 of them—was cruel. But I understood the government's reasoning. They'd become a threat to our society.

Sure there weren't that many. But there were enough. And they were a reminder of times when we, as a country, hadn't thought things through. We gave them citizenship too fast. We let them breed. We put them on pedestals and let them run up bills higher than some third world countries' GNPs. All in the hopes that they would teach us something worthwhile.

We were wrong. But we tried to deal with it. Until the virus. Seems it didn't become contagious until they hit their old age. Which I suppose was about three years ago because Mom was still alive. She'd joined one of those groups that was fighting for the aliens' rights. The groups were trendy, antiestablishment, lobbying and handing out flyers that exposed the plight of the homeless creatures. No real dangers. And they made no real progress. Like the hippy she'd been in her youth, my mom was still looking for causes. But she'd never chosen them well.

It took us awhile to trace the virus back to the aliens, but when we did, the outcry began in earnest. They infected everyone they came into physical contact with. No one was dying, but it was a nasty disease. A rash. Not a normal, small rash, though, this was one that went wherever there was hair. And the hair fell out. It wasn't pretty.

Even the groups like my mom's didn't want to be around them. Suddenly the advocates were silent.

The solution? That took a while. We had the ship. The ship could fly. But we didn't know what its fuel source was. Didn't know how far it could go. So we never took it up. Couldn't risk American lives. But we could use it to ship the aliens back to wherever it was they came from. Surely the aliens originally had enough fuel to get back—not our aliens, but the smart aliens, the ones who built the thing.

I know, the logic was faulty. I think we all knew,

but no one wanted to talk about it. The politicians told us it would all be fine; scientists showed us graphs and numbers; and soon the aliens were being rounded up. Groups, at first. Not families, because the aliens didn't have families. But after their downfall from the media pedestal, they started hanging out together in groups of four and five. And that was how the police originally found them—in camps on the rivers, lean-tos in the forest, cardboard homes in the alleys. They knew what was happening, knew they were being repatriated, but they didn't fight back. One thing the aliens had never done since coming here was fight. They were sheep. Stupid, hairless, shrunken-headed sheep. And I felt sorry for them.

We don't usually go to the park. At least not to the grove, where the whores and dealers spend their evenings. But Cili needed to collect different kinds of fall leaves for a kindergarten project. It was daylight, a busy weekend, I had Mace, and it seemed as safe as it would get.

So out we went, enjoying the cool fall air and the adventure of braving urban danger.

The leaves were crispy beneath our feet, the scent of detritus and distant smoke mingling for a pleasant, sensual odor that reminded me of camping trips and meadows. I held Cili's hand as we walked deep into the grove, ignoring needles and beer cans that hadn't yet been cleaned up by the groundspeople. We were determined that this be nature. The sky was bright, the day unseasonably warm, the sound of a nearby stream lulling us into easy smiles as we stooped and collected leaves by the dozen, as well as some interesting moss and one unsuspecting frog.

"Can I keep it, Mommy?" Cili whined and begged until I eventually agreed.

"Great! We can stop on the way home and buy a cage and some food and leaves and everything."

I had no idea what frogs ate.

As Cili ran to collect some pebbles by the stream, I heard him. Stealthy little fused feet crackling the brittle leaves.

I pulled out the Mace. "Cili!" I yelled. "Come here, hon. We have to be going."

I tried not to panic, tried to pinpoint the direction from which the sound had come.

"Cili!" and I saw her come running to me just as the alien stepped out of the trees and turned as if to go.

They collided in a heap of alien, child, and detritus. "Get away from her!" I yelled as I quickly covered the distance between me and them.

Cili was giggling, the alien struggling to disentangle himself from her. "Sorry," he said over and over. "My fault, my fault."

I grabbed my daughter and dragged her a safe distance away, glaring at the creature.

"I'm okay, Mommy," Cili insisted, but all I could think of was the virus.

"Stay away!" I told the alien though he made no motion toward us.

"Please don't tell," he begged, his beady eyes as wide as they could go. "Don't tell. I'm not hurting anyone."

"The virus," I hissed, looking meaningfully at my daughter.

"I'm clean," he said. "Really."

I turned, dragging Cili with me, and ran from the grove.

"Please don't tell," he yelled from behind me.

We cleared the park, and I had my daughter safely buckled into my Suburban. I looked at her beautiful blond hair and hoped she hadn't been infected.

"Mommy," Cili broached as we pulled out of the parking lot. "Can I have an alien?"

"No, of course not. An alien is not a pet."

"But they'll take him away. You wouldn't let them do that, would you? And he's so alone. He's got no family, Mommy. No one to take care of him."

"He's a grown-up, honey."

"That doesn't mean he doesn't need anyone."

"Cili, stop it. You can not have an alien. Understand?"

She nodded, silent.

After a few minutes of pouting, she busied herself with looking through the bag in her lap. "Pretty leaves," she said as she spread them out on her legs, the alien seemingly forgotten. "And moss. I like the moss. So will Kermit," she smiled excitedly as she remembered, and reached into her pocket, where she'd left the frog. I waited for her squeal of delight.

"Oh, Mommy," she said, instead nearing tears. "The froggy's dead."

Great, I thought. Just great.

Cili brought him home, and I can't say that I was all that surprised. Her attachment to the aliens had grown by leaps and bounds since the first time she saw one up close and personal the previous week. She kept insisting he needed someone. Everyone needed someone.

Bob was his name. Bob the alien. Can you imagine? They weren't a very clever species.

Cili was supposed to be at a friend's house. I had no idea she was so devious.

When I came home and found Bob, I had some serious thinking to do. He had been telling the truth about the virus at least. I'd given it a day, long enough for any signs to make themselves apparent. But none came. If he'd been a carrier, we'd both be starting to itch before then. If he'd been a carrier, I would've turned him in.

I stared at Bob, his silly, hairless, trusting face, his oversized clothes, clunky shoes.

"They'll take me away," he said, simply. What could I do?

Bob lived with us for a month. He couldn't cook, didn't clean, never quite understood the concept of locking the doors when we left, but he was sweet. He watched a lot of television and played with Cili until she ran out of energy. I didn't even know that was possible.

At first, I let Bob stay because I couldn't be a hypocrite to my daughter. She knew I didn't agree with the round-ups. I'd even written letters to the editor about the camp where they were keeping all the Bobs (as we came to think of them).

After a while, I grew to like Bob and his strange ways. He made me smile when he padded around a corner to ask once again how to turn on the VCR, his hairless little head lowered in embarrassment, flipper-hands folded politely in front of him. He regaled us with stories of the beautiful ones from his own planet—their shiny pates, their flat feet, black, beady eyes.

Cili was mesmerized by him. She hated to leave him even for a moment.

As time passed, I started to wonder what it was like to live in this strange place. So few like him, adored for a while, then detested. A stranger in a strange land just trying to do the best he could with what he had. All the other Bobs he'd left behind. A whole life left behind. Yet he never complained.

"It'll be okay, Bob," I overheard Cili telling him one day. "Some people are hard to find. Like my grandpa. No one knows where he is."

"Is anyone looking?"

"Sure. Someone must be."

"I bet it's not the government. If it was the government, they woulda found him by now."

"I won't let them find you, Bob," she promised. "You won't ever have to go away."

And I believe she would've done anything to keep Bob safe. I think I would've taken the risks myself in the end. I truly came to like our Bob. He wasn't bright. He got confused easily. And he was a slob. But he tried to be a good . . . person. He was kind to us, and helped us in the small ways he could.

But it wasn't our choice. After the fines were announced, after the first of the refugees were taken at gunpoint, the people who were hiding them jailed,

Bob left. We woke up one morning and he was gone. And I understood. He did it for Cili.

The day has come. Bob and the rest of the aliens are going home. It took over a year to round them all up. I followed it all closely, hoping for news of Bob, hoping there wasn't any. I read every article about every apprehension. I followed all the Bobs' stories and silently rooted for them. Once, I even prayed.

But by Cili's eleventh birthday, they were all in the camps, all awaiting departure, all milling slowly about, mending their worn clothes, shining one another's bald heads. Once, I thought I saw Bob, but I couldn't be sure.

The news reports made them look happy, but I think it's just their size and lack of hair. They don't cry, they don't complain, so how would we know?

The ship has been powered up to the best of anyone's knowledge. So Cili and I made it a sort of vacation to come out here to Florida. And maybe some private detective work. I'm glad we're here to watch all the Bobs take off and to say our good-byes.

Cili still doesn't understand. I don't try and make her. I don't want her to.

We stand in the early morning light, listening to the reports along with hundreds of others who have come to see the aliens off. Some are crying, some cursing, some have signs that say "Aliens go home" or "We'll miss you" or simply "Good-bye." One says "Diane, will you marry me" and I can't even imagine what that guy is thinking.

The camera crews surround us, microphones squealing, lights bright in our faces, soaking up this personal moment. I shield Cili as best I can. She's crying. I let her.

By the time the countdown has reached three, the sun has risen and its light turns the strange oval ship into a silhouette. Quite surreal.

The crowd is hushed, reverent when the announcer proclaims "We have lift-off" and we watch the oval rise slowly, slowly, slowly into a bright orange sky. It hovers for a moment and I think of those 208 visitors cramped into a space of less than fifteen-hundred square feet. I think of the graphs and the numbers, the theories and the rhetoric, and I hope they will make it home. I hope their home will welcome them.

"Is that it?" Cili asks as the ship bounds out of sight. "Is Bob home?"

"Yes," I tell her, hoping she won't hear the way my voice rises in false confidence. "All the Bobs are home."

"And us?"

As the sun shrinks and the sky turns blue, as cars begin to honk at one another and drivers curse as they try to get back on the interstate, I take Cili's hand. We walk slowly back to my new truck with the daisy on the tailgate and the paisley on the bumper.

"What about us?" I ask as I heft her into the passenger seat.

"Are we going to find home now?"

I pull a crumpled piece of paper out of my pocket. I run my finger along the three possible addresses, smoothing them out. "Yeah," I smile at her, my voice regaining its music. "Let's see what we can find."

SCRIPTURE GIRL

Edward Lee

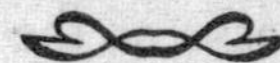

SMITH DIDN'T KNOW WHAT HE WAS DOING. HE DIDN'T care. *Maybe I'm an alcoholic,* he considered. *Maybe I'm just antisocial.*

He hadn't been to the Undercroft in over a year. The neighborhood tavern—it used to be his hangout. An under-the-street joint made of original Federal-period brick, all full of dark, veneered wood and polished brass. And people.

It had changed, he supposed, in his absence. Smith ordered another pint of Tucher Fest. *Or maybe I'm the one who's changed,* he surmised. He didn't know anyone here tonight, and he didn't want to. A new crew behind the bar, new patrons—neo-yuppies—and even new music—contemporary pop. Used to be on any given night he'd walk in and instantly be surrounded by friends; he'd even gotten lucky here on more than a few occasions. *Jesus,* he thought. *I don't even* have *friends anymore.*

"Do you believe in out-of-body experiences?" a voice to his right inquired.

Smith turned his head. It was a woman sitting on the next stool. Pale red hair, slightly mussed. Jeans. A tacky, billowy jacket. Smith couldn't quite fathom an answer to her question.

"I, uh," he began.

"Or remote-viewing?" she asked. "Or trance-channeling?"

"Well, uh—"

She took a sip of her drink: soda water. "Do you believe in God?"

Why this roundhouse of questions from a woman he'd never met? Smith skirted it all, extending his hand. "My name's Smith," he introduced.

Her hand felt particularly hot when he shook it. Or maybe it was just on account of the weather outside. The state had just been through the worst ice storm in a hundred years, and record low temperatures remained. Or—

Or maybe her hand felt so hot because Smith himself had turned cold of late, from the inside out.

"I'm Ruth," she said. "I haven't seen you here before."

"Well, I—" Smith began, but the rest withered. *I used to come here a lot,* he felt inclined to say. *But . . .*

But what?

But I lost interest in people. I lost interest in the world.

"I've been real busy lately," he said. "Haven't had much time to get out."

"I haven't been busy enough, I guess that's why I'm here," was her odd reply. The tenor of her voice seemed just as odd as her words. She sounded slightly sinusitic, and though she spoke at normal volume, her words seemed muffled, drained of clarity. "Well, do you?" she asked again. "Do you believe in God?"

"Sure," Smith accommodated her. *And I believe in Santa Claus too. And the Tooth Fairy.* But these thoughts were really just excuses stained by mordancy. Smith, in truth, didn't know *what* he believed in, if anything at all.

"Then why are you here?" this girl, Ruth, asked next. Her eyes darted to his beer, quick as a mouse pointer. "The body is a temple of the Lord."

Smith was hard-pressed not to gape. "What?"

"Someone explained it to me once," she went on. She was looking at him as she spoke, while Smith stared forward at the mirrored bar racks. "When you put good things into your body, you pay homage to God. But consuming bad things is the same as vandalizing a church, throwing rocks at the stained glass windows, spray-painting curse words on the altar."

Smith practically finished his beer and lit a cigarette simultaneously. "Interesting simile," he commented. "Can I buy you another drink—a soda water, I mean?"

"Okay."

Now what had he done *that* for? Smith had stopped prowling bars for women ages ago, and even if he hadn't, there were far more sightful prospects here than Ruth—the bar was lined with them, in fact. A pretty blond here, and foxy brunette there. They came here by themselves and always left with someone. It wasn't hard. But this girl, this . . . Ruth . . .

Her pale red hair, cut short, looked disheveled. The entirety of her did, in fact. Scuffed sneakers, frayed jeans, the fluffy lavender jacket with minute tears and flinty smudges. She looked ragtag, she looked poor. Her pale-gray eyes could've been puddles of drab water, like the ice-melt in the gutters outside. Perhaps that's why she'd piqued his interest. In all this downtown singles' bar glitz, she seemed as out of place as he.

"Do you believe in life after death?" she asked, looking intently at the side of his face.

"Sure," Smith said with the same disregard. But why wasn't he talking to her—talking to her *really? Stop being an asshole for once in your life,* he directed himself and sipped his fresh beer. "I mean, I don't know. I guess as I get older I become less prone to believe in things I can't see."

"Do you believe, for instance, that the words coming out of my mouth right now are real?"

"Well, of course."

"But you can't see them."

"I could with an oscilloscope."

She didn't hesitate. "Do you believe in the magma at the core of the earth, then? You can't see that."

"Well, I—"

"And you just said that you believe in God." Her flat eyes seemed to be boring into him. "Have you seen God?"

Smith shrugged.

"Life can be very beautiful," she continued, "if we

look at it closely enough. I think the problem with both of us is that we don't look at *ourselves* closely enough."

Now Smith frowned. How on earth would she know what *his* problems were? But then there came another consideration. Smith didn't really know that himself, did he? But it was interesting, the simple way she'd slotted them both into the same category. *Misfit,* he thought. *We're both misfits.*

"We're both looking for something," she said. "But we don't even know what that might be, do we?"

What did that mean? She was arcane, elusive, but Smith sensed very clearly that she wasn't trying to be.

Then she said, " 'Whosoever goeth into the world with no heart, leaveth blind.' "

So that was it. A religious zealot? She must be, quoting scripture. But why here of all places, in a bar?

" 'How much better a thing it is to strive and fail than to never strive at all, for those who never strive at all are like ripe fruit on the tree gone to rot, or a seed never fallen to the soil. The seed will not grow' "

Oh, man, what have I gotten myself into? he thought. *I've gone and picked myself up a holy roller. Next she'll be trying to sell me a carnation, or recruit me into some Christian cult.*

Suddenly he felt split down the middle, one half wanting to mumble some excuse to leave. But the other half . . .

What was it?

For the first time, he looked hard at her. The pale-red hair, the puddle-gray eyes. She sat stiffly on her stool, as if discomfitted. She seemed slender to the point of minor malnutrition, and the unpainted nails on her small hands were bitten down to the quicks.

" 'There can be no greater offense than to turn one's back on the gift of life that He giveth thee, for there can be no value in a life not lived.' "

He looked at her face. No, she wasn't pretty, no in any conventional sense, but she was . . . something else. Her face looked lusterless yet somehow hot with some kind of energy, her lips pale yet full. She wore no earrings, the tiny lobes not even showing evidence of piercing. A woman completely unadorned, undecorated, untrimmed in this world or ersatz glamour and veneered appearances. Quite like Smith himself.

He knew nothing of religion beyond his college classes, and as far as "holy rollers" went, he couldn't be more intolerant. Small peeps of people pushing answers on him to questions he had no concern for whatever. He knew he should get out now, go home, go back to the pallid porridge of his life. What he needed least of all was a fanatical ball and chain dragging him down. *Yeah, get out of here,* he convinced himself. *She's a nut. She probably watches Jimmy Swaggert.*

But as he continued to look at her, he felt more and more adhered to this place. With no forethought at all, he began to imagine her naked. She'd be skinny, of course, pale as milk, with only diminutive packets for breasts, and her ribs showing. Suddenly Smith was stricken by the most peculiar arousal. Her thinness—her *haggardness* close to the point of emaciation—seemed to hide something so vital he felt jealous. She was burning for something—his acceptance, perhaps, or perhaps something even more simple, a quest to allay her loneliness. Smith actually couldn't imagine what it was she burned for, but whatever it was it made her more interesting, more scintillant, than other women in the bar, the dressed-up, pretty dolls, so many women thrusting themselves forward as attractive furniture in their tight dresses, their lipstick and makeup, their spurious women's-magazine faces.

Shit, he thought.

Her knee touched his, but he felt certain this was not deliberate. She seemed oblivious to the fact that her body was making contact with his. With any other girl in the bar it would be an overt come-on.

Did Ruth's knee feel . . . hot?

At once Smith felt smothered, a claustrophobe in a broom closet. "Look, Ruth," he said. "You wanna go for a ride or something?" But this question he instantly regretted; it sounded way too forward, like saying *You wanna go fuck?* This was not his motive at all. He just wanted to get out of here. Hastily he added, "Or go to a different bar?"

"Okay," she agreed. "This place isn't for us, is it?"

Smith rolled his eyes. "On me," he said when she produced and opened a big clunky purse. He couldn't help but notice stray cash showing in the purse's maw, tens and twenties, even fifties, crumpled there as if stuffed. So he must be wrong, at least about her being poor. When he paid both their bar tabs, she distractedly said, "Thank you."

The cold air bit him in the face the instant they left

the tavern. West Street looked like the main drag in an abandoned city. "My car's right over here," he said, swallowing cold air. She calmly followed him to the graveled sidelot, her dowdy sneakers popping over the ice-encrusted rocks. Smith pinched his collar together but the frigid air slid down his chest nevertheless. *God, I hate winter,* he thought, but then he realized that he actually hated all the seasons. Shivering, he opened the passenger door of his car—a clay-red '67 Malibu, a clunker—and joked, "The Lamborghini's in the shop."

"What's that?" she asked plainly and got in.

"Never mind." He actually laughed, closed her door, then got in on his side. The steering wheel felt like a ring of ice; his breath condensed in front of his face. The engine grated, slugged, then started up, loud as a tank. He gunned the gas, impatiently snapped on the heater. "Sorry," he apologized. "This big land yacht takes a few minutes to heat up."

"Oh, I'm not cold," she replied. She seemed to be looking curiously around the inside of the car.

Smith pulled out and headed down West Street. He wanted to get the engine going, to get some heat. "Wanna beer?" he asked, awkwardly reaching in back to the bagged six-pack. "Oh, that's right. You don't drink." He paused. "The body is a temple of the Lord."

"Uh, yes. That's right. Alcohol takes the edge off one's spirit. Drinking it is like—"

"Spray painting curse words on an altar," Smith recalled. He would've chuckled but that might offend her. Actually he admired her abstinence. He crooked the bottle of lager between his legs, opened it with a church key while guiding the car with the other hand, expertise honed by sheer experience.

"It's so pretty out tonight," she said rather distantly. Her eyes seemed wide, gazing out the windshield in a wonder almost childlike.

"Yeah," Smith agreed. He supposed it was. The stars in the sky seemed over-bright, like chips of luminous gems. In the distance the eerie blue light turned the dome of the State House into an azure skull.

"'The Lord made the world in beauty, for all mankind to behold.'"

Ho boy, Smith thought. *I picked a winner this time.* It just seemed so contrary. *When you pick a woman up in a bar, she's not supposed to quote the Bible, is she?*

And that was exactly what he'd done, something he *hadn't* done in longer than he could remember. He'd just picked a woman up in a bar. And—

What now?

Smith faltered. Was he actually nervous? He knew his motives weren't really sexual, so what were they?

When he sipped his beer, he found that it had turned to slush in the cold. He lit a cigarette more to distract himself than anything else. The scenario was building up to something. He didn't know what he wanted it to be.

"So where do you feel like going?" he finally commenced. The moment of truth. What would he do if she said *How about my place?* Or, worse, *Your place?*

"Someplace pretty," she answered.

Smith struggled with the request. That could mean

anything. But at least she didn't want to go to another bar, and that relieved him. *Someplace pretty. Shit.* The city looked evacuated, routed by plague. Closed shops and drab, cramped rowhouses passed on either side. The City Dock would be jammed with cars and drunks, and the Historic District was now little more than a ghetto. *The water,* he thought then, amazed by his ingenuity. Yes, any woman would think that was pretty. *Go to the bay-road, take her out to the water.*

"Let's go look at the water," she said as if psychic. "I'd like to see the stars sparkling over the water."

Smith raised a brow at the coincidence. *Tell me I don't know what women want,* he joked. He turned off the Circle, then gunned it up onto the bay-road.

At last, the heater was producing heat. He made to turn on the radio but then pulled his hand back. She would want to talk on the way, not listen to dismal music. "So what do you do, Ruth?" he asked.

"Nothing, really." Her finger raised, pushed a stray strand of hair back behind her ear. "Just searching for what I want. Like you."

Smith spared the reply that came to mind. Testily he wanted to ask her why she kept implying that he didn't know what he wanted out of life. That this was true didn't even matter. *She's a weirdo,* he thought. *So let her be weird.*

"I want to have a regular life, you know."

"Okay," he said, "but what's your definition of 'regular'?"

She glanced down in her lap, at once seeming forlorn. "It's different for me. I *have* to. At least you have a choice."

Smith winced through his smile, the cigarette sticking out of his mouth. "What do you mean?"

"Never mind," she fairly whispered.

Icy patches on the black road looked like scabs of white crust. Black-flecked ridges of snow lined the curbs.

"I want to see something pretty," she said. "Something nice. I'd like to go look at the water."

"Relax," he assured her. "That's where we're going. I know a great place."

"Is it pretty?"

Smith rolled his eyes again. "Sure. It's this little place right on the bay. We can see that stars and the water and the green and red lights blinking on the big navy antenna network."

"Lights," she said and recast her eyes to her lap. But she seemed to be smiling now. She seemed happy with Smith's choice, and for some reason he suddenly wanted to do something that would make her happy.

But why would he want that? She was a stranger essentially, someone he'd just met, and someone he didn't even know if he liked. A holy roller. A nutcase. And then it dawned on him just how weird this whole thing was. *She's a whack. She's not even good-looking. And here I am driving her to the bay. Christ . . .* Why had he pursued this in the first place? Had something drawn them together? And if so, what?

We're both misfits, he repeated his earlier conclusions. *I guess I'm a weirdo too, just a different kind . . . .*

At least that was something, and something was better than nothing.

For the last few years he'd felt all too content in his

withdrawal from the world and in his swelling antisociability. He felt at home in it now, and, no, not once did he ever believe he was missing out on something, as Ruth's subtle remarks seemed to imply.

Or maybe I'm just blind, he thought back to the first scripture she'd recited. *Blind and don't know it. Can't see anything and don't want to.*

He stilled the morose thoughts. They were almost there. When Smith reached down to tap an ash in the lit tray he noticed her purse perched between her feet. It was still open, still showing the crumpled bills stuffed there. How naive could she be? Some guy she just met in a bar? There were a lot of guys out there, especially in this town, who wouldn't think twice about conking her on the head, taking her money, and raping her to boot. *It's a fucked-up world. A dirty, grimy, ugly world full of evil people . . .* Or maybe she was just absent-minded. Who knew?

But Smith noticed something else. In the purse. Even in the chopped moonlight, and the feeble light from the dash, he could see the book. A thick black-covered book wedged in the purse amid the errant, crumpled bills.

A Bible.

Ruth was an amalgam. *Goes to bars but doesn't drink. Has a purse full of loose cash, and a Bible.* Yes, she was a puzzle with red hair and blanched-gray eyes. *With my luck,* Smith considered, *she's probably an escapee from some mental ward, a runaway loonie.* And though he'd thought this in jest, the idea quickly lost its humor. Unkempt, tackily dressed, wearing sneakers, for Christ's sake. Not what you would call the typical gal about town, making the scene . . .

How did I ever get myself into this? he wondered. The bay-road wound on, narrowing into darkness; Smith, in fact, felt like the long stretch of road looked: desolate, unfeeling. He wondered what *she* felt. He wondered if she'd ever been in love. Then: *Have I?*

The query seemed to hang. But he was certain he had, in the dim past. Women had loved him, and what had happened? Smith crushed their love up into pieces with his own two hands, like something made of papier mâche.

What is love anyway? he challenged himself. *Is that what she thinks I'm looking for? Is that what she thinks I'm blind to?*

" 'Those who know not love,' " she suddenly said, " 'are like the fishes in the deepest sea. But those who know love are forever blessed, for God is love.' "

"Hmm," Smith replied. "You're a Bible scholar?"

"No, just a student of life, you might say. And I guess I'm not doing very well in my studies."

Well, don't feel bad, honey, Smith thought, driving on through the dark. He knew little of the Bible: just a couple of theology courses he'd taken as electives well over a decade ago. He'd gotten nothing out of the classes, save for the extra white elephant credits he needed. But one line did come to mind, just now, from Ecclesiastes: *Wisdom exceedeth folly, as far as light exceedeth darkness.* Was that what Smith's life had reverted to? Folly? Darkness?

He felt he must say something, lest the entire night turn sour as curdled cream. Most of the stuff she was spouting sounded like Old Testament, the stilted, barren stuff. He remembered another line. " 'The multitude of the wise is the welfare of the world.' "

But all she did in response to this was look at him, as if perplexed. Perhaps his recital had been too obscure, a scripture she hadn't heard. It figured; it was just more of Smith's luck.

"We're here," he announced. The trees broke. At once they were driving the edge of the bay-road, winding around. Smith remembered the area; years ago he'd driven a girl here one night. A picnic spot sat elevated just off this estuary of the bay. Smith pulled into the same log-bordered parking enclave now, switched off his lights. The engine murmured, the heater gusted warm air. He didn't dare turn the motor off—they'd be shivering in minutes.

"Look," she said, astonished.

Through the windshield they could see the water, its low saline content sufficient to keep it from freezing. It looked like a great, black mirrored pane before them, reflecting stars.

"And . . . look," she said, jerking her gaze. "You were right!" In the distance, a network of blinking green and red dots of light could be seen, like odd stars themselves.

"It *is* beautiful here."

"I told you," Smith said.

He leaned back in the bench seat, lit another cigarette. The reflection of a high moon lay blurred on the bay's surface, wavering slightly as the water rippled sluggishly. The vision tranquilized him, like a stiff shot of bourbon. The stars bore such clarity they seemed like swirls of phosphorescent spillage.

"Tell me about yourself," Smith bid. "I really don't know anything about you, except that you read the Bible."

A pause unreeled. Was she hesitant, nervous? But, oddly, she answered, "We all have a purpose, don't we?"

Smith shrugged. "I guess."

"So what happens if we don't fulfill that purpose?"

We die unfulfilled, Smith supposed, but that would be too nihilistic to voice. Why couldn't he think of something positive to say? "Maybe we're not supposed to know what our purpose is," he said. "Maybe fulfillment isn't as easy to see as we think."

Her mouth seemed to purse in confusion. "I just know," she nearly whispered, "that I'm not doing what I'm supposed to be doing."

"What's that?"

"What everyone else does, for all of history. 'The Lord gave life, and the purpose to create life. In new life there are joyous hearts, but man findeth no purpose in seeds unsown.' "

What was she implying? How absurd? She couldn't be that old. *What's she worrying about?* Smith wondered. *Her biological clock? She's probably not even twenty-five.* A few more lines popped into his head. " 'Give me children or else I die'? 'Be fruitful and multiply'? That the kind of thing you're talking about?"

But Smith's heart lurched when he took another glance. She lay back against the seat, her head lolling, her mouth hanging open like a trap. Drool shined on her chin. *Holy shit!* Smith exclaimed, reaching out. Was she diabetic? Epileptic? *Christ almighty!* He touched her shoulder, nudged her around. "Ruth? Ruth?" *Fuck!* He rummaged through her purse, hoping to find some bottle of medication, but all he found instead was her heavy black Bible and the tufts of cash. No wallet. No housekeys.

And no medicine.

The moment froze in his fright. *What if she dies? What if she's dead now?* He jostled her some more, eyes wide on her lax face. Her head rolled as though her neck were broken. But then he remembered what she'd said, one of the very first things back at the bar. Something about trance-channeling, out-of-body experiences? *Christ. What a fuckin' nightmare this turned out to be . . .*

But just as Smith was preparing to back the car out and take her to a hospital, she slowly revived, her eyes fluttering.

"My God, are you all right?"

"God?" Her eyes fluttered. "Wh— oh, I'm sorry. I scared you."

"You're goddamn right you did," Smith struggled not to yell. "Are you all right?"

"Oh, yes. I was just . . . thinking."

Thinking? This was awful. This was a big mistake. What on earth had been on Smith's mind anyway?

"Look," he said. "It's getting late. Maybe I better take you back now—"

She nearly lurched forward. An urgency—even a terror—seemed to crimp her face. "No!" she blurted. "Please—"

Smith's stare lengthened. How could he ever figure this out? How could he ever figure *her?* He tried to think of something else to say, but before he could—

What the hell is she doing n—

She shucked off her tattered jacket. Her bitten fingers raised to her blouse—

You've gotta be shitting me . . .

And she began to take off her clothes.

All Smith could do was sit there slack-jawed and watch her strip. She did so falteringly, her nervous fingers traipsing like a spider from one button to the next. The ragtag blouse slid off. Then she popped the metal snap, awkwardly arranged herself, and struggled out of the frayed jeans.

"I'm not very good at this," she muttered.

You ain't kidding, Smith thought, but by the completion of the thought, she was nude. She'd worn no panties, no bra; Smith noticed an unruly pubic patch and faint tufts of fur under her arms, and this he found mildly arousing for whatever reason. At first she seemed backed against the passenger door, a tiny, timid sable backed into a corner by poachers, her nakedness the predation. The moonlight reverted her to a nervous, tinseled shadow.

Then she began to slide forward, across the expansive bench seat, toward Smith.

She was so *white,* but he saw now that what he'd previously observed as a ghetto pallor he'd mistaken for refulgence, for lambency. Odd as she was, he found her strangely beautiful.

She'd ridden him, so to speak, had clumsily sat on his lap, facing him, after he'd just as clumsily gotten his pants down. Mechanically, at first, he'd tried to do the things he thought he was supposed to do: stroking her, kissing her. But she'd tremored at these touches, sealed her lips to his attempts to kiss. *She has no idea what she's doing,* Smith realized. *She's never been with a man, she's never even been kissed . . . She's never done this before.*

The suspicion was verified a moment later. When she straddled him, and guided his penis to enter her, she shuddered, stiffened in a wince of pain, and repressed a cry.

Smith felt some gossamer *thing* break inside of her.

Aw, Christ, he thought, wincing himself. *She's a virgin, and she didn't even tell me.* Most men, he knew, entertained the fantasy. *Popping a chick. Busting a cherry.* But Smith, of course, wasn't most men. Nothing could make him feel more vile than taking a woman's virginity under such fly-by-night circumstances. He'd just torn open her womanhood, in the space of a blink. It was supposed to be something special, wasn't it? It was supposed to be something reserved for high school love. But what choice had he had? She'd been the one, not him. She'd come over and simply sat on him, and that was it. No time for debate, nor consideration. No time to even talk to her about it.

"I thought it would hurt more," she whispered. "I guess that's why I was so scared."

"You should've told me," Smith complained as his pulse rose. She felt so hot inside. Her arms wrapped around his head. The seat creaked. He could feel her blood trickle warmly between his legs.

What have I done? he thought.

The minuscule breasts pressed flat to his chest; he girded her waist with his arms, could feel her skin-tight ribs. His eyes peeped just over her right shoulder, and he could see the moon's sphere reflecting atop the water. It's light bobbed, then seemed to smear as Ruth continued to ride him. More of her blood trickled but she didn't seem to care—she seemed very focused now, on pins and needles to get him to come—she didn't seem to mind what must be extraordinary discomfort. She held Smith's head tighter, then, her wan breath gusting. Then they both nearly shrieked at the same time.

How proverbial, Smith thought a few minutes later. He lit a cigarette, his shirt and jacket had never been removed, yet his pants remained ludicrously bunched at his ankles. She lay back too, back on her side, still naked and tinseled silver by the moonlight. Smith needed time to get his breath back, and still more time to think of what to say now. He wanted to say something nice, something sincere, or at the very least something phony that would make her feel good. But perhaps there was nothing to say at all.

" 'Blessed are the fertile,' " she said in a parched voice. Her eyes slitted in some arcane satisfaction.

But Smith thought, *Blessed are the fertile?* It sure didn't sound like anything Jesus had said during His Sermon on the Mount.

" 'For the fertile,' " she continued, " 'bring forth more to share the blessings of God.' "

Smith's brow furrowed in confusion.

"Thank you," she said. "I have to go now."

Smith nodded, exhaling languid smoke. "Sure. I'll take you back," he said, still flummoxed over the entire situation. "Let me get my pants back up—"

But that wasn't what she meant; she meant she had to go *now*.

"What are you doing?" Smith exclaimed, his cigarette bobbing.

The dome light winked on and freezing air exploded into the car.

She'd just opened the door . . . and was getting out.

He reached for her, his pants still preposterously bunched around his ankles. "Get back in the car! What kind of a nut are you? You'll freeze to death out there!"

But she wasn't listening. She was walking instead. He could see her through the windshield: walking naked in the frozen wind toward the water. And then—

Smith gaped.

She was walking not into the water, but *on top* of the water.

Toward the spherule of floating moonlight.

The light blurred then. Smith's gaze yanked to the left, and he saw the real moon, far off over the trees in a position that couldn't have possibly reflected off the water.

The orb of light rose, then blossomed, and Smith was momentarily blinded.

And then the light was gone, and so was Ruth.

He remained staring, blinking, too dumbfounded to even reach over and close the door to shut out the cold. Yes, she was gone.

He looked down into his lap, to find his hips covered with something much thinner than blood. It was like pink water on his thighs, and glistening in his pubic hair.

The motor continued to purr. Not only had she left her clothes, she'd left her purse, which he picked up at once. When he rummaged through it he found what must be hundreds of crumpled dollars. And there, wedged into the middle of it all, was her Bible.

Smith opened the book, squinting in the dome-light.

God, he thought.

It was a Bible, all right. But its scriptures, tacked along each nearly translucent page, were printed in no language he had ever seen.

THE THRESHOLD OF BEYOND

Stephen Mark Rainey

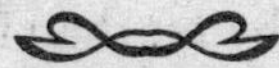

THE WRECKAGE WAS STREWN OVER AN AREA TWO miles long and a quarter of a mile wide, the largest intact piece no bigger than a car door. Most of the debris had been burned to cinders, for, despite having only a small amount of fuel on board, the plane had ultimately exploded with a fireball that could be seen more than twenty miles away. Far from the crash site, hundreds unaware of the tragedy thought it extremely odd that thunder should accompany the light snowfall that had begun a short time earlier.

Threshold Air Flight 1890 took off from Chicago's O'Hare at 7:55 P.M.—on time—on Saturday, December 21, bound for Providence via Newark. The evening's last flight into Theodore Francis Green State Airport was Captain Zack Taylor's first time on the route; for that matter, it was his first flight with Threshold ("From New England and Beyond!" as the airliner's slogan boasted). He'd been forced to sign on with the smaller carrier after his previous employer, one of the major airlines, had cut its routes down to the bare minimum in an attempt to avoid filing for bankruptcy for at least another few months. Taylor was accustomed to flying L-1011s and DC-10s, and now, cramped in the cockpit of an MD-88 that had obviously seen more than a healthy share of commutes since its last washing, he was forced to wonder if the company maintained the crucial workings of the plane any better than its external surfaces.

The plane was loaded with holiday travelers, and traffic at Newark had been as busy as Taylor remembered ever seeing it; but somehow, ATC had moved the flight right through the system with scarcely a minute's delay, even though many of the bigger carriers were announcing waits of several hours. The weather had been fairly cooperative on the flight from Chicago, with only a few unpleasant bumps around 20,000 feet. New England would likely see snowfall tonight, judging from the clouds gathering up and down the Atlantic coastline, but it probably wouldn't hit until sometime after they'd landed. Fortunately, Taylor didn't have to fly again until late tomorrow afternoon, on the return trip to Chicago. By then the airports should be all cleared, unless the clouds brought a blizzard with them, and the forecasters didn't expect that likely.

Descending to flight level 10,000, leaving behind the lights of Bridgeport—what few could be seen through the broken clouds—the airliner shuddered briefly as it passed through an area of turbulence. Ellen Chaves, the head flight attendant, had warned Taylor that they were carrying more than the usual number of nervous passengers, and one woman in particular screamed shrilly at the slightest bump; there had probably been a few anxious gasps just now, followed by relieved giggles as soon as the ride smoothed out. Fortunately, in his almost seven years with his previous airline, Taylor had never experienced an actual in-flight emergency, and he'd only once had trouble with a disruptive passenger the flight attendants couldn't handle. Cynically, he wondered if, after "downgrading" to Threshold, his good fortune could hold out.

He had to credit the airline with one thing—its training program had been at least as thorough if not more so than any of the major carriers', and in its twelve-year history, it had suffered only one accident of any consequence: a crash at LaGuardia in 1989, a 737 whose left wing landing gear hadn't locked down, causing the plane to skid off Runway 13 into Flushing Bay. There had been fatalities, but the majority of the passengers survived. Sadly, the captain and crew did not.

From his headset, a crackling voice caught his attention: the controller from Boston Center. "Threshold 1890, adjust altimeter to 28.65. Check Providence ATIS on 124.20."

Taylor replied affirmatively, and tuned his com radio to the Providence airport information channel. The recorded broadcast informed him that winds were out of the west-southwest with up to fourteen knot gusts, with an 1,800 foot ceiling, overcast; that meant a variable, twenty-degree headwind and very limited visibility. Traffic at PVD was relatively light, and they could expect to land in about twenty minutes on Runway 23 left.

Taylor's copilot, Lawrence McPherson, now flew this route frequently, but had only been with Threshold a few months himself. A native of Providence, Mack was going home now and would get to spend the holidays with his family, as he didn't have to ship out again until New Year's. Out of the corner of his eye, Taylor saw McPherson's face crinkle in annoyance.

"Did you hear that?" Mack said, pulling his headset back. "I'm getting a mess of interference here."

"No, mine's okay."

"Maybe it's the set. Or maybe it's just my ears. I've been hearing weird stuff all night."

"Oh? You hadn't mentioned it."

"Figure it's the weather. But if yours is fine, we ought to get the set checked out."

The plane shook again, but this near to their destination, they couldn't climb to a more comfortable altitude. They'd have to make the best of it. Taylor's eyes ran over his instrument panel, confirmed that fuel flow, engine pressure, airspeed, and altitude all read normal. Flying in cold weather could be very taxing, and after being based in Atlanta over the last few years, he'd have to get used to these New England winters.

Only partial corpses were recovered from the wreckage; not a complete body could be found by the searchers, and it was all too plain early on that no one could have survived. The plane had come down in a wooded area outside of Pawtucket, and even though rescue crews had arrived within minutes, reaching the crash site took almost an hour. Several columns of smoke, each spaced nearly half a mile apart, indicated the distance the plane had traveled, smashing through trees and scattering pieces of itself like dead leaves in its wake. Fortunately, no ground dwellings had been in its path, so casualties were confined to those on board the aircraft.

Providence Approach Control would guide Flight 1890 north and east around Providence, taking them on a wide path over North Scituate, Lonsdale, and almost to Attleboro before turning them southwest toward the airport. Mack kept having trouble with his headset, and Taylor had had to ask the controller to repeat his last message as a sudden crackle of interference over his own set drowned the distant voice.

"This is bad," Taylor said, looking down at the still distant but expanding warm glow amid the gray ocean beyond the cockpit windshield. "The weather's starting to pile up, I'm afraid."

"My head is killing me," Mack said, rubbing his temples. "Just came on suddenly. Of all times."

"Here," said Taylor, reaching into his pocket and taking out a packet of ibuprofen. "I'm getting to be a junkie on this stuff."

"Thanks," Mack said. He had a partial can of apple juice left from dinner and chased the pills with the remainder. "Man, will I be glad to get home tonight."

Providence Approach broke in over Taylor's headset. "Threshold 1890, turn right heading one-two-zero and descend to four thousand. Contact tower at intercept Whitman radial two-seven-zero."

"Roger, approach, leaving ten thousand, descending to four thousand," Taylor replied, throttling back and gently nudging the wheel forward to begin a 2,000 feet-per-minute descent. Airspeed read 245 knots. As the plane nosed down, Taylor turned the wheel slowly to the right, wincing as the aircraft entered a pocket of low pressure that caused it to drop several hundred feet in a couple of seconds—like having the carpet pulled out from under your feet, he thought. He compensated for the change quickly enough, but he imagined the nervous woman in the back of the plane must have just let out a loud one.

Directing the plane on a course to intercept the radio signal from the Whitman VOR, Taylor suddenly found that the OBI dial, with its to/from indicator to show the plane's position relative to the station, was not activitated. The nav radio was properly tuned to frequency 114.5.

"What's this?" he said, tapping the dial with his fingertip. "What have we got here?"

"Damnation," said Mack, checking his own dials that mirrored Taylor's. "It's out. And no radar!"

Taylor saw that the upper dial, tuned to the ILS, or localizer frequency to guide the plane down to Providence's Runway 23, had also gone blank.

"Hey," said Mack, looking up and pointing out the windshield ahead of them. "What the hell's that?"

The Pilot of the MD-88 had informed both Providence Tower and Boston Center that they were encountering lots of radio interference, but there had been no reports of trouble with any of the other systems before the plane went off the center's radar scopes. However, the final messages from the crew had been garbled, and until the flight recorder could be recovered, there was no way to determine exactly what had happened in the cockpit in those last few minutes.

A number of witnesses in the Pawtucket area had reported seeing the plane break through the clouds on its approach. Some said they couldn't hear its engines; others said they knew it was in trouble because it was coming in so low. However, some witnesses claimed to have seen a second aircraft, and believed that there must have been a mid-air collision.

The only wreckage, however, had been from Threshold Flight 1890.

Taylor gazed at the shape that had materialized in the black canopy above the seething, lead-colored masses below. Unknown miles distant, the thing appeared as a cluster of vaguely glowing spheres, descending very slowly. It was not blinding, but the surrounding haze diffused its light so Taylor could not discern any surface detail—if, in fact, the thing were solid.

"Is that a plane?" Mack said, then answered himself: "No, no, it isn't."

"I don't think so. Maybe some kind of reflection on a cloud. Light from the ground coming through a break in the lower layers."

"Yeah," Mack said with a nod. "Doesn't seem to have a cohesive shape."

That much was true. The mass appeared to fluctuate in size, one moment compact and dim, the next swollen and more brilliant. Just before reaching the first overcast layer, where Taylor expected it to perhaps merge with the vapor and dissipate, the cluster suddenly halted its descent, hovering motionless in mid-air, its lights still oscillating rhythmically.

Taylor and McPherson exchanged glances. "Boston Center, this is Threshold 1890, do you have any traffic at flight level ten-zero in our two o'clock position?"

A voice responded in Taylor's headphones, but crackled in and out unintelligibly. He repeated his query, only to receive the same garbled reply. A call to Providence Tower yielded identical results.

"Damn it," he muttered, turning his attention to the inoperative instruments. "We've got to get this cleared up fast. Keep trying ATC."

Taylor looked over the instrument panel, verified that only the radio systems appeared to have failed. The fuel gauge indicated they had 5,000 pounds left, enough for about an hour in the air. Glancing up, he saw that the strange congeries of lights remained stationary above the clouds, seemingly remaining at a constant range. It was either extremely large or flying at a synchronous airspeed and heading—or both.

"Nothing," said McPherson, rubbing his temples. "I'm not getting anything now. Not even static."

"Providence Approach, this is Threshold 1890,"

Taylor said into his mike, forcing his voice to stay steady. "Are you reading? Come in. Please."

Dead air.

"Hang on," McPherson said. "I think I'm getting something. I'm on 135.4."

Taylor listened as McPherson called in again. A faint whisper rose in the headset, incomprehensible; it might not even have been the controller's voice. Tuning to Providence Tower on 120.7, he said softly, "Providence, this is Threshold 1890. Do you copy?"

He heard the same ambiguous whispering on this frequency, realizing that he could not possibly be hearing Providence Tower. This was a weirdly modulated rushing sound, similar to ocean breakers, but with an erratic rhythm, like but unlike the pattern of speech. A second hiss joined the first in strange harmony, seemingly far in the background.

"Oh," said McPherson suddenly, looking up through the windshield. "It hurts."

"What's the matter?"

"It's in my head."

"You going to be all right?"

"I—I don't know." He pulled his headseat down and let it loop over his neck. "Christ, it hurts."

Now the sounds over the headset took on the quality of a distant, inhuman chorale; eerily sentient, yet random in its meter, with more and more distinct, separate tones merging into a single rush of kinetic sound.

Taylor noticed that McPherson's eyes clamped together; his face was suddenly whitewashed by a flare of light from the sky beyond the windshield.

Suddenly he saw that the OBI dials had come back to life. But the needles that centered on radials emanating from directional beacons on the ground whipped wildly back and forth, the to/from indicators flashing back and forth in meaningless alternations. And outside, the glowing spheres had fused into a single, brilliant mass like a nighttime sun, and had begun to move—on what appeared to be an intercept course.

The one thing Zack Taylor had never felt on board an aircraft was helplessness. Even when riding as a passenger, he felt comfortable in the air, knowing exactly what was happening in the cockpit, understanding each structural creak when the plane hit turbulence, gauging thrust by the sounds of the engines. For the first time in his life, Taylor knew exactly what that poor nervous woman in coach must feel every time she boarded a plane—deep and total impotence in the face of something incomprehensible. For her, the very concept of a machine weighing hundreds of tons lifting off the ground, supported by a cushion of air; for him, something occupying a sky where there should be only clouds and perhaps another airplane. Something brighter than the moon, and at an altitude that meant it posed a threat.

"Taking evasive," Taylor said, whipping the headset from his own head. "Hold on, Mack."

He banked the plane sharply to the right, knowing the maneuver would shake up the passengers; and he had to hope that no nearby traffic lay in their path. Certainly, any other planes in the vicinity would see this intruder, and hopefully, somebody with an operable radio could alert traffic control to what was happening.

As the plane veered to starboard, the light swung out of view, but a brightening highlight on the nose just outside the windshield gave ample evidence the object persisted in its rapid approach.

A moment later, darkness returned to the night outside, except for the warm glow of Providence beneath the murky, vaporous canopy below. Leaning to his left and looking back through the side window, Taylor saw no trace remaining of the object.

The cabin door opened and a shaken-looking Ellen Chaves stepped inside, brushing back a lock of blond hair that had fallen over her eyes. "What's going on? Was that a plane?"

Taylor shook his head. "We've got problems here. I want you to keep the passengers calm. Tell them we've got bad weather and we're trying to go around it. Just don't let them panic. Make sure they're all wearing their seatbelts."

"What the hell is happening?"

"We just had a close encounter."

For several seconds no one spoke as the reality of his statement settled upon them. Ellen's eyes betrayed her growing apprehension, but she cleared her throat and nodded, aware that the responsibility for maintaining order in the cabin fell upon her.

"We've got some radio problems. We're going to have to stay up here until we get it sorted out. We're not in immediate danger, provided we don't have any more, uh, unusual company. You all right?"

"Yes. I'll take care of everything, Captain."

"Thanks," he said, uncomfortable withholding from her the dire truth of their predicament. "Keep the faith."

With a concerned glance at McPherson, Ellen returned to the cabin, and Taylor could hear the rise of voices greeting her as she opened the door.

Checking his instrument panel, Taylor confirmed everything still functioned nominally except the radio systems. Then turning his attention to McPherson, he received another shock—for his copilot had gone deathly pale, his breathing short and rapid. His eyes had rolled upward, and his hands, lying in his lap, trembled violently.

"Mack!" Taylor leaned over and touched McPherson's wrist. His pulse throbbed furiously, and his skin felt cold and clammy. "Mack!"

McPherson suddenly sat up, eyes wide, seeming fully alert. He gazed curiously at Taylor for a moment, then his features changed gradually into a taut grimace of fear. He whispered something Taylor couldn't understand until he leaned close.

"What is it, Mack?"

"All in one. It's coming through the all in one."

Taylor and McPherson exchanged anxious looks. "What is it? What does that mean?"

"It's coming."

Intuitively suspecting that something from outside might be affecting the copilot, Taylor turned to look out the windows. At the moment he could see nothing. But a glance at the instruments assured him that something more had gone amiss: the inertial compass read 180 degrees; the magnetic compass showed 25 degrees. Often during tight turns the magnetic compass could not correct itself as quickly as the inertial system, but by now it should have recalibrated.

McPherson gazed pitifully into Taylor's eyes. "Why? Why me?" Then, his head lolled back, and a hoarse moan rose from his throat.

Outside, a warm glow spread over the white nose of the plane. Taylor's eyes whipped back and forth, seeking the source of the light, but the night sky revealed nothing.

"It's above us. Jesus, it's right on top of us," he whispered to himself.

The comforting rumble of the engines suddenly wavered. Stuttered.

And fell silent.

"Oh my God," Taylor gasped, watching his instrument panel go dark before his eyes. "We're going down."

As the layer of clouds rose to meet them, Taylor looked at his copilot. McPherson's body had gone completely rigid, his lips pulled back in a Sardonicus grin, eyes bulging from his sockets, their rims blood red.

"It's here," came McPherson's voice. "Ia."

Behind them, the cabin door flew open and Ellen Chaves stumbled inside, admitting the frightened cries of the passengers. And the flight attendant screamed, the sound driving deep into Taylor's brain, crowding out any remaining rational thought.

Her scream was not a reaction to the sight of the ground rushing toward them, but to the thing that now occupied the copilot's place; a thing which bore no resemblance to Lawrence McPherson. Or to anything that any living human being had ever witnessed.

Forensic teams were eventually able to identify all the human remains from the crash. All, that is, except for the copilot, Lawrence McPherson, of whom no trace could ever be found.

What was found among the wreckage shocked the original team at the site so badly that some of them refused to take part in further investigating the accident. Unfortunately for them, no evidence to substantiate their claims of finding something "terrifying in the extreme" among the remains could be recovered by subsequent investigators; a few rescuers on the scene had hesitantly intimated that a bizarre, chitinous "appendage," lying in the vicinity of the ruined cockpit, withered and disintegrated only a few minutes following its discovery.

No official explanation was ever offered for the tracks, as some insisted they be called, leading away from the site through the woods in the direction of Providence. Indeed, while the series of deep indentations in the earth might give the impression of a deliberate stride from something quite large and heavy, traveling on multiple, irregularly shaped limbs, anomalies arising from such devastating impact could not only be possible, but, based on precedence, anticipated.

Sadly, the true cause of the crash of Threshold Flight 1890 died with the passengers and crew of that ill-fated aircraft. The flight recorder, when recovered, offered no clues whatsoever; in fact, its examination merely added to the mystery that still enshrouds the accident, for despite the mechanism's appearance of functionality, when played for the investigators, the recordings provided only three-quarters of an hour of total silence, as if the aircraft and all those aboard had never existed.

THE GLASSY APES

Tracy Knight

For J. N. Williamson

ROCKING BACK AND FORTH, THE MAN IN THE WHEELchair knuckle-scrubbed the crown of his enormous head.

It was late evening in the Golden Ark Nursing Home. Echoes of moaning residents mingled with the sickly sweet smells of antiseptics and clabbered flesh: a sensory symphony of the end; an aria of endless waiting.

I sat down in front of him and opened his file on my lap.

Name: Marcus Stillson. DOB: 1930 (?). Diagnoses: Severe mental retardation; hydrocephalus; paraplegia.

Mr. Stillson's room was bathed in shadow. The wistful winter moon glowed against him, angling in through the large window he faced. Outside, colossal snowflakes swirled and whipped, dancing madly with the shrieking wind. Unblinking, Mr. Stillson gazed out over the flat Midwestern landscape and its unbroken, mounting snow.

The hydrocephalus was his most striking quality. His hairless head was huge. Undoubtedly he was born with the condition and had never been treated with a shunt to redirect the accumulating cerebrospinal fluid. Thus, as a child his skull had enlarged with the increasing cranial pressure, adjusting as best it could. We humans are, if nothing else, graceful adjusters to the vagaries of life. Somehow, we get used to it all.

I pulled my legal pad to the top, then looked closely into his pale, delicate face. Amazingly, unlike most with his condition, the skull's enlargement hadn't caused a widening of the nose; it was a button nose, almost cute. His mouth was similarly small, a pencil sketch on his face. His ears were tiny. Only his moist, dark eyes were in proportion to his massive head.

"Mr. Stillson?" I said more loudly than necessary.

No response. He continued rocking, scrubbing his head, staring out the window.

I reached up and gently touched his shoulder.

He jerked his face toward my hand, grimaced, and tucked his chin into his chest. A string of drool emerged from one corner of his mouth, lengthened, then fell into the lap of his bathrobe.

Not much chance of conducting a proper psychological evaluation, I thought. Making a human connection with him would be impossible.

I scribbled a few observational notes, then copied the diagnoses just as they appeared in the file. Nothing to add to this case. It was a formality; evaluations were required whenever new residents were transferred in from a state institution.

I stood up slowly and, before I turned to leave the room, I impulsively leaned down next to Marcus Stillson's ear and whispered, "I can relate to you, my friend. I've lived my life in the shade, watching and waiting too long, just like you. And now, you know what? The doctors tell me I have three months to live. That's right, cancer. Sometimes it's hard not to just let go of the rope." I tried to stop talking but couldn't. "A depressed, hopeless psychologist. That's rich, isn't it? Kind of like a dentist with yellow crud on his teeth. Well, spending time with good people like you has made my life better. Take good care, Mr. Stillson. Godspeed."

"Dr. Everett?"

Startled, instantly feeling self-conscious, I turned to face the administrator of the nursing home, Loretta Bender, who stood in the doorway.

"Here a little late, aren't you?" she asked with the frail smile that had always beguiled me. For the ten years I'd worked with Loretta, whenever I was near her I felt like a schoolboy scuffing a shoe against playground gravel. Forever wanting to be closer, I'd never found the strength or resolution to traverse the intangible membrane that seemed always surrounding her, protecting her subtly sad face from the world.

Now things were different. Now it was as if I viewed her across a vast abyss. I wished I had known her better while I was truly alive.

But to one already resigned to loneliness, to death, regrets are as meaningless as hope.

I shrugged. "Things have been busy at the private practice. I didn't want to keep you waiting for these reports."

"But it's a Saturday night," she protested. "And it's snowing something fierce."

Again, a shrug. I'd become adept at shrugging. "It's either this or spending an evening at home with nothing but brandy and boredom to keep me company. It's worth the risk of getting snowed in."

She ran her hand through her long chestnut hair. "You're a sweet man, Arthur. We appreciate you here." She paused for a moment and seemed to examine my face more carefully than usual. "Are you sick or something? You haven't been looking well lately."

"Just old age creeping up on me," I lied. "Turned fifty-one last week."

"Still just a kid," she said, winking. "Barely a lap ahead of me."

A faint, flickering part of me wanted to say something else, something about us maybe having dinner together someday or seeing a movie or taking a walk or just sitting down and talking.

It quickly extinguished. All these years, she'd never given any indication of hearing my indirect, clumsily spoken invitations for us to spend time together. But I could hardly blame her. Since my wife died fifteen years earlier, and even before, I'd never been one to speak clearly when it came to matters of the heart. I was a man who'd lived life selflessly, honorably, consistently, but as if I was always waiting for something. Waiting.

Maybe that's why I felt so at home in Golden Ark. Maybe that's why swimming in the pains and joys and struggles of strangers had been such an attraction to me: part of it was compassion and a true ability to help my fellow human being, sure. But part of it was envy.

And now, understanding that, it was too late.

"Anyway, this was the last evaluation," I said. "They were all pretty straightforward."

"I'm glad you're here with Mr. Stillson. I need to talk to you about him." She laid an index finger across her lips and narrowed her eyes. "One question, Arthur: Did you call Dr. Oleas and have him discontinue Mr. Stillson's Thorazine? Before you'd even examined him?"

"Yeah, this morning, when I first reviewed the records. I've never seen a file with so little information in it. No social history. No psychiatric history. The strangest thing is that this fellow'd been on Thorazine since the drug was invented, yet I found no indication it was ever needed. No evidence of psychosis or agitation."

"Well, you know the institutions. Used to be they'd put everyone on a major tranquilizer just to keep them quiet."

"Then I'm happy Mr. Stillson found his way to Golden Ark. I only wish we knew more about him."

"He's quite a mystery," Loretta agreed. "He was first institutionalized in New Mexico in the late forties. We're not even sure how he ended up in

Illinois, but he's been in umpteen facilities across the country."

I gestured toward Mr. Stillson. "Has he been rocking like this since he arrived?"

"No. Just for the past couple of hours."

I nodded. "Thorazine's wearing off. We'll keep a close eye on him tonight. It may turn out he needs the medication after all. But let's just wait and see. He at least deserves the chance."

"I think we're going to be forced into a quicker decision." Loretta clearly felt troubled about mentioning this. "Mr. Stillson's guardian demanded that we hold an emergency meeting tonight. He'll be here any minute."

"Why?" I asked. I'm sure I was frowning.

"He called me this afternoon to see how Mr. Stillson was doing and blew up when I told him the doctor had stopped the Thorazine. He wanted to get here right away but the snow's drifting, roads are closing. He just called again from his car phone. He's on his way."

"Seems to me the guardian should be happy we aren't drugging Mr. Stillson into oblivion."

Just then, Loretta's eyes widened. All expression melted from her face as she took a step into the room.

"What's the matter?"

She didn't answer. She didn't have to.

A man wearing a dark green parka appeared behind her, a man with a pit-bull body, an ice-white crew-cut and a scowling face latticed with deep age lines.

He held a revolver at Loretta's back.

"I'm Captain Blake Munroe," he said in a rough voice damp with phlegm. "I'm Mr. Stillson's guardian."

Neither Loretta nor I could respond immediately.

"How long has he been off the Thorazine?" he asked.

"Since this morning," I answered, hearing the tremor in my voice. "About twelve hours."

He twisted his head, disgusted. "Dammit! Then I have to kill him."

He pushed Loretta into the room. She fell against me and I held her there, close.

"Who are you?" Munroe demanded.

"Dr. Everett. I'm the consulting psychologist."

"You're the fool that ordered the medication stopped?"

I nodded.

"I should kill you, too," Munroe said.

"What's this all about?" I asked, arms spread. "What do you want?"

"I've been his guardian for nearly fifty years, mister." A strained look fell across his face. "I *know* what he needs. And now . . . now you've ruined it, ruined everything. I can't stand here and bullshit with you. He has to die. Those are my orders."

Munroe took a step toward Mr. Stillson.

Mr. Stillson had no awareness of what was going on around him. He continued to stare out the window into the galaxy of snow, ever rocking, ever scrubbing his head.

I had to act. To stand there and do nothing, I knew, would haunt me the rest of my life. All three months of it.

Munroe pressed the gun's barrel against Mr. Stillson's gigantic head, puckering its soft flesh at the temple.

"Don't!" Loretta cried. "You can't kill him! He's helpless!"

"Lady, if you want someone to blame for this, blame yourselves."

I let go of Loretta and dived toward Munroe.

My shoulder struck him just below the knees. He toppled sideways.

The gun fired as it flew from his hand. Sparks leaped off the ceiling fixture where the bullet hit.

I scrambled to the gun, grabbed it, stood and, still trembling, said, "Stay right there, Captain Munroe!"

Munroe slapped the floor with contempt. "Jesus Christ! You really don't see, do you? You don't understand what you've got here."

"What have we got?" I asked, trying to mask my anxiety. "Tell me."

"Look at him! You think he's just some worn-out old man? He's not human!"

I looked briefly toward Mr. Stillson, then back to Munroe. I was mystified. Munroe was the one who seemed inhuman to me. "The man's totally disabled. He's lived with more problems than most of us in this building put together. But he's human."

I felt Loretta's hand on my back. "Arthur," she said, "I'm going to call the police."

"Please do."

She left the room. Her footsteps echoed down the hallway.

Munroe chuckled as he stood. He brushed off the front of his parka. "You don't know what the hell you're talking about. Listen here: I've been his legal guardian since the forties. I *know* him. We retrieved him from the crash of an extraterrestrial spacecraft."

"Spacecraft?" I exclaimed. "As in flying saucer?"

He nodded, steely eyes riveted to me. "He was the only survivor. He's been in the army's care ever since. It didn't take us long to figure out that the only way we could maintain a semblance of control was if he was on Thorazine and kept away from people as much as possible. That's why he's been in institutions and nursing homes all these years. It was our best option until we figured out how we could best learn what we needed to know without endangering everyone. And now . . . you've done *this*."

As I listened to Captain Munroe, I became convinced that the Thorazine had been prescribed to the wrong person. I expected him to begin foaming at the mouth any moment. My best bet was to keep him talking until the authorities arrived. "So tell me, Captain Munroe, what's this terrible thing that's supposed to happen when the medicine has completely left his system?"

He seemed oddly relieved that I'd asked the question, as if he'd heard a whisper of belief in my tone. He sat down in a chair, crossed his legs and interlocked his fingers over one knee. His voice became almost friendly. "What happens? Honest, I can only guess. What we've discovered is that the aliens are . . . *absorbers* of some kind. At first we thought they'd come to Earth only to explore: you know, flybys, collecting soil samples, the occasional cattle mutilation. We were okay with that. But it's more.

Memories, feelings, they extract them from us. We're not sure whether they harvest human experiences for study or simply . . . digest them; maybe both." He paused, and I thought I saw the first traces of tears shimmering in his eyes. "Without the medication, we couldn't stop him from feeding. Hell, even when he's snowed on Thorazine, the process manifests to a small extent. So we placed him in mental institutions and nursing homes, where plundering memories and feelings would do the least damage, maybe even help the people he was near. If we'd kept him alone, he'd have died. Starved. And we could never learn. . . . But now it'll be out of control. I have no choice but to kill him. Believe me, I wish that wasn't the case. I can't tell you how much of *my* life he's taken from me, having contact with him all these years. He's fed on me, too. I've lost a lot. And now . . . it was all for nothing."

"So they take our memories and feelings," I said, eyes flicking toward the door, praying Loretta would come in any moment accompanied by a uniformed man more accustomed to tense standoffs than I. "That still doesn't answer my question. What do you think will happen when the medicine wears off?"

"We have no way of knowing. He's never been off of it since the early fifties. He might be too weak to do anything by now; then again, we might have a feeding frenzy on our hands."

"What about . . . the other aliens? Aren't they looking for him?"

Munroe shrugged wearily, suddenly looking like the seventy-year-old man he must have been. "Until we put him on the Thorazine, his people's crafts filled the skies. Then they were gone—poof!—just like that. We're not sure whether they're trying to punish us by withdrawing . . . or if we've scared them off by keeping Stillson captive. Who knows? Maybe they're off bugging someone else."

"What have you hoped to learn from him?" I asked, becoming increasingly intrigued with Munroe's delusion.

"How we can control and use the absorption process. *We* could decide which feelings and memories were taken. If we could do that, imagine the implications! We could siphon off overwhelming memories, overpowering emotions. Look, you can appreciate that. There'd be no more depression or anxiety in the world."

"No passion, either," I said. "Perhaps no love."

Loretta appeared at the doorway, panting. "Phone lines . . . they're out . . . the storm."

I turned in her direction for only a split second, but that was enough.

Munroe jumped to his feet and slammed the full weight of his bullish body into me. The force of it threw me backward into a wall.

He snatched the gun from my hand and shoved me to the floor.

Then, in a startling blur of motion, Mr. Stillson flew from his chair, landing on legs I thought had long been useless. Incredibly, he vaulted at least six feet into the air, sailing over Captain Munroe's head.

Mr. Stillson lurched from the room, bone-thin arms and legs flailing wildly, massive head bobbing left and right, bathrobe trailing behind him like a cape.

Munroe exited the room in pursuit. I grabbed Loretta by the arm and we followed as quickly as possible.

Mr. Stillson was running toward the front lounge impossibly fast, his gait a bizarre, spastic ballet. He leaped against one wall, sprung off with all four limbs, then jumped toward the other wall, repeating his strange performance.

Munroe raised his gun and aimed at the moving figure.

"Don't!" cried Loretta. "You'll hit a resident!"

Munroe paused, and Mr. Stillson took a final long leap, somersaulted twice, then darted sharply right, into the lounge—out of sight!

The lights went out.

We were swallowed for the moment by absolute darkness. Terrified, Loretta and I held each other tightly.

Then the emergency system near the ceiling came to life, small spotlights splashing errant angles of white against the walls.

Captain Munroe stood, seemingly mesmerized by the eerie illumination, staring blankly, gun at his side.

We ran the rest of the way to the lounge and were just in time to see Mr. Stillson—whoever or whatever he was—hurtle his ghostlike body to the front picture window. He stood there a moment on wavering legs then raised his arms, pressing his thin fingers against the frosty glass.

The front window of the Golden Ark Nursing Home imploded, shooting millions of glittering shards across the room. Immediately the icy wind invaded, carrying a cloud of thick snow.

Captain Munroe turned toward Loretta and me. "You see?" he shouted, barely audible above the bellowing wind. "You *see?* He's losing it!"

Losing what? I wanted to ask Munroe but too much was happening. Chaos filled the hallways: sounds, sights, smells, the frigid squall, the flying snow.

Suddenly, Munroe's arms fell limply to his sides. His mouth went slack as he dropped his pistol.

He slumped to the floor and began seizuring, body convulsing, palms pressed against his temples.

I stood watching. Waiting. So unsure of myself and what I should do I couldn't move.

"What's happening?" Loretta screamed above the clamor. "Arthur!"

I opened the door to an empty resident room to our left. "Go in there, Loretta, please! Stay put until I come for you!" I half-pushed her inside and closed the door.

A legion of voices rose up, swelling in the hallways, merging with the blizzard's roar.

Whatever this was, it was happening throughout Golden Ark.

Mr. Stillson remained immobile before the shattered window. Snow and ice were accumulating on him. I wanted to go to him, to pull him to safety.

But then I peered down each hallway.

And I saw the source of the cries.

Residents were spilling out of their rooms, stumbling down the darkened hallways. Some walked erratically. Others whose legs had given way squirmed, thrusting their feeble bodies to and fro as they made their way toward the lounge, toward Mr. Stillson, toward me.

Timeworn voices screamed and thundered. A Greek chorus of pain and fear.

Whatever powers I possessed—to empathize, to understand, to swim in the oceans of others' lives—were useless.

I ran to Munroe, knelt beside him and shouted, "What's happening? What can I do?"

His wandering eyes focused on me. Reining in ragged breath, he said, "Memories. He can't hold them any longer. They're spilling out of him. Back to their owners! Oh my God!"

I gasped. Munroe's face was starting to stretch like rubber. His lips pressed together in a tight grimace that widened and widened more. Red fissures, steaming, appeared on his forehead and spread across his face. His skull cracked and split apart. His head lost shape, blood and brain matter appearing at the surface of the skin, finally dribbling and then pouring from his face.

Residents' screams whirled around me, a tornado of sound.

I rushed down the hall toward the pharmacy, thinking I might locate injectable Thorazine. I no longer doubted much of what poor Munroe had said. I tried to leap over the stumbling and slithering residents.

A man so old he looked like a skeleton emerging from a flesh cocoon advanced to me and grabbed the front of my shirt. I looked into his red, rheumy eyes. They were shining with unfocused, unbridled terror.

"I remember!" he cried. "I remember!"

Instantly I wasn't standing there anymore. I was

sitting on the front steps of an old farmhouse, hot breeze tousling my hair. I watch a young towheaded boy grab a kitten by the tail. It cries out. He lifts it over his head, pauses, then batters it against the sidewalk again and again and again, its skull splintering, ribbons of blood and brain arcing up across the noonday sun. The boy turns to me and laughs and laughs and laughs . . . then

I pulled away from him.

"I remember!" he cried, slamming his fists against his head.

Before I could respond, an old woman, eyes ablaze, pushed toward me and grabbed my tie and yanked me close to her and I was

reaching for a young girl's back. She stands before a crumbling, ancient well, something in her arms. Thunder crashes overhead. Lightning throws our shadows to the ground. The girl turns to me, weeping, and shakes her head. Releasing the bundle, she steps back, averting her eyes. I bend forward and see the newborn, arms spread, legs kicking, sailing downward, downward . . . splashing . . . stillness . . . then

a tremoring hand grabbed my ankle. Looking down I saw another ancient man, face screwed into something raw, and I was *patrolling with a platoon at the edge of a tiny village. Ahead I see the soldier. A naked teenage girl kneels before him. Laughing, he points his rifle at her. Tears stream from her eyes. "Please . . . meester." He pulls the trigger. Crimson blossoms from her forehead and she collapses into the mud. The soldier turns to me and winks . . .*

"God forgive me!" cried the man on the floor.

Images and sensations reeled through my brain and body. I shook myself free of all the trembling, grasping hands, clapped my own hands against my ears to shut out the screams.

Munroe had said that the memories were spilling out of Mr. Stillson. Apparently they were finding their way back into the minds of those who'd lived them. And yet they could not be integrated by their original hosts. There was no room for them. Life had healed around the empty places.

So now, the homeless memories were leaking out with my touch, leaking into me . . .

Cracking and splitting sounds pierced through the roar of the invading snowstorm. Several residents collapsed and fell still as their heads were rended, faces and skulls splaying, ripping apart from the force of unbearable memories . . .

Standing on tiptoes I looked down the hallway, squinting into the half-darkness. The pharmacy was at the other end. There was no way I could reach it through the teeming mass of Golden Ark residents. Further, if my understanding was correct, injecting Mr. Stillson with Thorazine would likely be of no help now. The damage was done. The stolen memories and feelings had escaped.

And yet, why was *I* not affected?

I turned and ran toward the room where I'd left Loretta, dodging the residents, slipping and sliding through the snow and ice gathering on the floor, the bodies. If nothing else, perhaps I could save her, save the one person I'd wanted to connect with but didn't, take her away from the madness, through the blizzard and to warm sanctuary. Somehow.

When I opened the door to the room, it thumped against Loretta's prone body. Her breathing was shallow. Her head tossed left and right like she was trying to throw off a dream. I reached down and put my arms around her, pulling her up to me and hugging her tightly, and I was

standing at the threshold of a child's bedroom. A large man in a soiled undershirt stands over the dead body of a little girl who lies in a fetal ball on her bed, blood pooling around her. He turns to me and shouts, "She wouldn't stop crying!" I feel a sob catch in my throat as he comes toward me, meaty fist raised. He strikes me hard on the temple. I crumple to the floor. "Elvin!" I hear myself crying. "Why are you doing this?" He ignores me, lifting his fist again. I crawl on all fours to the couch, reach under the cushion, pull out something and hide it beneath me. The man jumps onto my back and begins pummeling me with fists, then bangs my head against the floor, again and again. With great effort I strain against his weight, turn over.

I plunge a twelve-inch butcher knife up through the

bottom of his chin . . . pushing, pushing, until it's buried to the handle.

He topples backward.

"Oh, Loretta," I whispered. "So that's why you'd never let me close. God, I'm so sorry."

Then it hit me. I was still touching her and the images, the emotions, all of it had vanished.

Thin red lines appeared on her forehead. Flesh opened. Wounds, like tiny scarlet smiles, appeared across her face.

I gathered her in my arms and stood. Moving through the doorway and into the frigid hall, I headed for the lounge, pushing aside howling men and women as I went.

Mr. Stillson stood at the broken front window, arms raised, facing the blaring snowstorm.

I gently placed Loretta on the floor, then clamped my hands on Mr. Stillson's shoulders and spun him around to face me.

A layer of ice covered his face, his enormous head, his large dark eyes. I looked closely and saw three or four tears frozen on his white cheeks.

"What's happening?" I demanded, shaking him.

He flopped in my grasp like a puppet.

And then I heard him. Inside my head.

Starving. I am starving. I am weak. And alone. Frightened. They've left me.

"Take them back!" I shouted, feeling the rage of helplessness, crying myself now. "Take the memories back!"

I can't. They are gone. All these years. Too weak to

hold them any longer. I'm weak, starving, afraid. But I knew you would come.

He smiled. Ice crystals dislodged from their place on his lips and pattered on the floor.

"What do you mean?"

You do not remember me were the words he spoke inside me. And childlike, he rested his enormous head against my chest.

And the memory washed over me like a warm, uncaring surf.

I am three years old and we are on vacation. Daddy and I leave Mommy and Sis at the motel and hike into the desert. Soon, my little legs tire and Daddy carries me.

I am the first to see the crashed spacecraft.

"What is that?" I ask.

Every bit as intrigued as me, Daddy sets me down and takes my hand, walking with me to where a lonely family of brush stands huddled in the desert. Beside it is a silver craft shaped like a wedge of Mommy's pie, crumpled and smoldering on the sand.

Around it, four bodies. Small creatures. Large heads. Wide, dark eyes.

Two of the creatures are obviously dead, bodies broken and scorched.

The other two are alive. One is badly injured, writhing on the ground. The other scrabbles around the sand on all fours, in circles, like a fevered dog dying.

"Stay back, son," Daddy says.

I stand transfixed, tears welling in my eyes. I want to go to the creature, pick it up, carry it away to safety, nurse it until it's whole and well.

My father gets down on his hands and knees, moves closer to the creature.

A gunshot pierces the air.

"Stop right there or we'll shoot at you!"

Four men in army uniforms approach, pull my father to his feet.

One walks to the writhing creature. "They agreed they'd never land!" he shouts. He aims his rifle and shoots the creature dead.

Another army man kneels before the being who crawls on the ground.

I watch unmoving as the soldier locks eyes with it and seems to communicate silently. He becomes as pale as a winter moon. His lips tremble as he speaks. "I can hear its voice in my head. But it doesn't make sense. All I know is that they're here for more than exploration. They're . . . hungry—"

"What are you talking about, Captain Munroe?" screams the officer. "Our previous contacts with them indicated there'd be no interaction with humans."

"—and worried." Captain Munroe shakes his head. "They're worried for us. Something about wanting to extract our strong memories and emotions so we can continue to live. It says we can't live with everything we experience. Life is . . . too big for us."

Daddy comes over and puts his arm around my shoulder. His steady strength settles me.

The officer, increasingly agitated, begins stomping in circles. "We'll take them all in, figure this out later."

"But—"

"That's my decision, Munroe! Pick up that creature and take it to the jeep. You," he said, pointing to the

other soldiers, "gather up the bodies. We'll send more troops out to clean this place up."

Captain Munroe picks up the struggling creature and stands there, face sallow, as the other soldiers converge on the dead aliens.

The officer tells my Daddy and me that we are never to say anything about this day or we'll be killed and left in the desert where the animals will eat us and chew our bones clean.

Shuddering, Daddy nods and we turn to leave.

But before we do, I turn back. And lock eyes with the little creature.

In my head I hear, Will you help me?

I want to, *I think,* I want you to be all right.

We shall meet again. We are alike. We will help one another.

I promise, *I thought, love swelling in my chest for an odd little man who needed my love and understanding.*

"I promise." Saying it aloud, the memory splintered and I was in Golden Ark again.

Mr. Stillson's smile faded. *Then you will help?*

"Wait. I still don't understand. You use us . . . for emotional food? That's all we are?"

He slowly shook his enormous head. *We live for one another. We helped create you from the apes. Not only for us, but for you. Yes, it is true, your feelings strengthen us. But we didn't foresee—*

"What? What didn't you foresee?"

That your ambitions would be superior to your abilities. Your dreams greater than your realities. Your awareness larger than your lives. You are still apes—beautiful apes—but so delicate, so fragile. Without us to relieve you of intense memory and emotion, you would go mad. Some still do. Have you noticed what has occurred since my people stopped coming? Too much life within you all. Madness. Inside, instinctively, you blame us, knowing we are interested, knowing we could help. Some of you even dream that we come to examine you, concerned again. You need us.

"To take away our memories," I muttered, "the feelings you think are too much for us to bear."

You are already dying, Arthur Everett, I know that. You have shared in so many lives, so many memories. You are full. You can feed me. I can live. And perhaps my people will return for me.

Even a hopeless psychologist can recognize choice points.

I could relinquish my inner life to the alien, thus bringing back his race to draw off humankind's disturbing remembrances, knowledge, passions. Life would be safer, more predictable, manageable.

Or I could carry out Captain Munroe's orders to kill the alien, making the earth safe until the army—or whatever groups were interested in such things—correlated all its data on Mr. Stillson and discovered how to drain the emotions *they* chose.

I looked down to where Loretta lay dying, head fracturing, eyes roving independently of one another, shallow breaths scarcely visible.

It is time to help me. As you pledged.

"I will," I said, reaching with trembling hands toward Mr. Stillson. "I will!"

Mr. Stillson pushed himself against me and my body shivered as I made the choice to use the gift I'd possessed since I was that tiny boy in the desert.

I enfolded him in my arms, held his fragile body tightly against mine.

It felt like I was turning inside out.

I smiled.

And absorbed Mr. Stillson's life into me, as easily and surely as I had caressed the lives of so many people all the years of my existence.

He struggled for only a moment, briefly raising his dark eyes to meet mine. Understanding. Forgiving. Perhaps even proud.

Body quaking, my head immediately surged with a tempest of awareness, images, sensations: of Mr. Stillson's life, on the earth and off: his pain and loneliness, his dreams.

Mr. Stillson's body folded into the floor, dead. Emptied.

Neither the aliens nor the army would decide which memories and emotions were fitting for us to store and wrestle with, not just yet.

I turned around and surveyed the hallways. Many of the residents were dead, heads consumed by all of the things they'd done—or *hadn't* done—and tossed aside.

But others were alive, struggling on the floor.

I moved to them, one by one, touched them and drew memories into me: storms of sepia photographs, discarded psychic scrapbooks of a thousand lives.

Once done, the residents—relieved of the pain they'd given up to the alien and could no longer reclaim—arose and stumbled silently to their rooms.

I turned around. There was one thing yet to do.

I went to Loretta's side. She was alive, but barely. Great spilling clefts crisscrossed her head.

Sighing deeply, I pulled her close to me and—as she took her final earthly breath—I seized what inner life remained of Loretta Bender and prayerfully absorbed it.

With the fleeting time left before my death, I contemplate the choices I made, the life I created. And I see that it was good . . . or, at least, very human.

Considering the universe of facts and memories inside me, I wonder if I should reveal all I've learned of the aliens, their natures, their intents. All I know of our fates.

But no, I think. We clumsy earthlings, we fragile apes: we shall have to do as best we can to experience and endure every shred of the lives we live.

We at least deserve the chance.

So as my own life ebbs out of me, I do the one thing I've avoided all these years. Selfishly, I bequeath one gift to myself.

I close my eyes and let myself be enveloped and lifted up by the multitude of lives I bear, each one an everchanging, gorgeous nova.

Just above me, I recognize Loretta. Though she has no body, no mouth, I see that she is smiling.

And like a tattered autumn moth chasing a dying sun, I flutter after her.

Hopefully.

NOTHING AS IT SEEMS

David B. Silva

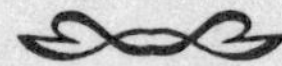

I

Will Cassidy doesn't talk about it anymore. Neither does his daughter, Chantal, who was eleven when it happened and is almost twenty-eight today. In fact, no one in Kingston Mills talks about it. But that doesn't make it any less their history.

II

For six weeks after Will Cassidy's eleven-year-old daughter Chantal had turned up missing, life had been a walk-through, a dreamlike, timeless state of drinking coffee to stay awake, of adrenaline pumping every time the phone rang, of trying to find an answer to the one question everyone was asking: How could this be happening in Kingston Mills?

Chantal's disappearance wasn't the first, though she was the second youngest, right after Bobby Cutler, who was only nine when he vanished. The very first person to disappear was Elmo Stanton, sixty-seven, who lived in a small one-bedroom apartment that sat over the Mills Hardware store on Main Street. Elmo had owned and operated the store for a good many years, as had his father before him and his grandfather before that. The Stantons had been one of the first settlers in Kingston Mills.

He had lost his wife to congestive heart failure three years before his disappearance, and though you could still find him at the Community Center on Bingo Night or at the hardware store during working hours, you didn't see as much of him around town as you once did. That was why it wasn't until midday on a Monday, when the store still hadn't opened, that someone finally became worried and a search was begun.

The second person to disappear was Emily Sanders, the town librarian. She had moved to Kingston Mills in 1972, having gone back to school and received a degree from San Jose State after her children had grown and left home. She was forty-two, married to a trucker who spent most of his time on the road, and her favorite activities outside of the library were karate (which caused her to make the long drive into Redding twice a week, usually after nightfall) and mountain climbing (the reason she and her husband had moved to Kingston Mills in the first place).

Emily disappeared on a Wednesday, two days after Elmo.

Robert Underwood had walked her out of the library that night, a little after it closed at nine o'clock. It was overcast, he remembered, because she had been disappointed in the absence of the stars. They were her reminder of her place in the world, she had told him. Like the stars, even though she was just a single flicker among billions, she had her own shine—we each had our own shine—and there was no telling how far out into space it traveled.

She was in good spirits that night, he said. Looking forward to spending some time with her husband, who was supposed to return the next weekend after a cross-country haul to New Jersey. Robert dropped Emily off at the front door of her house a little before nine-thirty, he guessed it was. He watched her go in, watched the lights inside go on, and then went about his way.

It was the last time anyone saw Emily.

The third disappearance came in broad daylight less than eighteen hours later. It was by far the most puzzling of them all, though there were at least half a dozen witnesses who swore they saw exactly what happened.

Two of those witnesses, Judy Landers and her husband Tom, were out running errands during Judy's lunch break from the five-and-dime, where she worked as a bookkeeper. They had stopped to pick up a pie from Sandy's Coffee Shop on Main Street, only four doors down from the Mills Hardware, where Elmo had disappeared. Out front, they had bumped into Lily Hanover. Lily, who had just celebrated her fifty-fifth birthday the week before by jumping out of an airplane at 10,000 feet for her first-ever sky dive, was excited about her second dive, which was planned for the upcoming weekend.

"You couldn't get *me* up there," Judy said. "Not if my life depended on it."

"Oh, God, you have to try it, Judy. Just once."

"I'd pee my pants."

Tom, who was holding the door open and only listening with half an ear, impatiently nudged Judy with his elbow. "Don't forget we still have to get over to the market before you go back to work."

"I know," Judy said. Later, she would confess that she had seen a glow in Lily that she had never seen before, and that in the back of her mind, she was actually wondering if maybe she should try a dive of her own, just for the boldness of it. But Tom was at her elbow and they were in a hurry and . . .

. . . and then Líly seemed to lose her feet all of a sudden. She stumbled backward toward the door to the coffee shop, the door that Tom was holding open, her arms whirling in the air like an acrobat trying to keep her balance, and in the blink of an eye, she was gone.

Judy remembered a moment of complete dumbfoundedness, when she looked at Tom to verify what she had seen and he looked back at her with an astonished, unbelieving expression on his face. They were both stunned beyond imagination. It wasn't until Martha Haberstein came running across the street, squealing with excitement that they finally snapped out of it.

"Did you see that? Did you? She was right there

one second and the next thing—*poof!*—she was gone. Like it was magic. Like one of those silly little coin tricks you can buy for a quarter over at the five-and-dime. Now you see it, now you don't. Absolutely incredible! My heart's pounding a thousand beats a second."

Martha had seen it.

Judy and Tom had seen it.

Two kids from over at the high school, playing hooky for the day, had seen it.

And there were others.

Lily Hanover had literally disappeared right in front of all of them.

And she wasn't the last. Three more people disappeared before Will's daughter joined the exclusive club. There was Adam Walker, twenty-eight, the postal carrier for Kingston Mills; and Teresa Saunders, who was raising two boys after their father had been killed while working for a logging outfit somewhere in Northern Oregon (her boys were staying with their grandmother, a little closer to town these days); and then there was David Winters, who had sat on the same stool at the end of the counter at the Stop Over Bar just outside of town for nearly every-day of his adult life.

They had all disappeared.

And then one day Chantal had joined them. She had taken the bus home from school, gotten off at her usual stop, and had been walking along the gravel road that ran perpendicular to Bakker Street at the northern edge of town. She was with her best friend, Amy, talking about what they were going to do for Easter vacation, which was only two weeks away.

Exactly what happened, Amy couldn't say. She remembered feeling a chill pass through them as if a sudden gust of wind had kicked up, only it was more like walking into an air-conditioned room in mid-August. It was almost as if they had passed through a wall of cold air, she said. Chantal zipped her jacket up and said something about how creepy it felt. And then she was gone.

Just like that.

One moment there, the next moment gone.

Will Cassidy heard about what had happened from his wife, Rachel, who had been home at the time and had heard it directly from Amy only a few minutes after the fact.

It might as well have been hours.

Chantal had joined the missing.

III

For the next six weeks, almost nothing in Will's life seemed focused. There was a soft, blurry edge to all the questions, to the day-by-day routines that had to be done, like it or not, to everything except Rachel. She had become the only clarity in the foggy haze, the only person who seemed to be able to navigate her way through what had happened and set about trying to do something to get Chantal back.

There wasn't much she could do. There wasn't much anyone could do. Because what had happened to Chantal, like what had happened to all the others before her, was a complete mystery.

Still, Rachel didn't let that get in her way. She had

posters made up with Chantal's most recent photograph—as well as photos of all the others who had disappeared—and used volunteers to distribute the posters throughout Kingston Mills, the neighboring town of Round Mountain, and most of the outlying areas of Shasta County. When she wasn't dealing with posters, she was on the phone talking to radio stations or newspaper reporters, to anyone who would listen, to anyone who might help to get the word out.

Will had not been as strong as Rachel. The night of Chantal's disappearance, he had returned from a trip to Chico, where he had spent the day at the Chico State Library researching a feature piece he was doing for the *San Francisco Chronicle.* Rachel had met him at the door with the news.

She had cried openly that night, freely, telling him more often than he cared to be reminded that she didn't think she would know how to go on if anything ever happened to Chantal.

Will didn't know, either.

And he didn't want to think about it.

He had never felt so helpless in his life.

IV

Several weeks passed, and then Bobby Cutler turned up missing.

Bobby, nine, who walked out of the five-and-dime after buying a pack of baseball cards, had disappeared less than a block away. Once again there were witnesses. And they all told a similar story, the same kind of story that Judy and Tom Landers had told about Lily Hanover's disappearance. Bobby had simply walked into a nothingness and out of existence.

Whoosh.

That fast.

That mysteriously.

And though no one mentioned it, everyone was thinking the same thing: Bobby would not be coming home again. None of them would be coming home again.

V

Will had begun to spend his evenings at the Stop Over at the edge of town. It was a little after eleven as he sat at the bar, nursing a scotch that was the second of two shots he would down all night. He had never been much of a drinker. Chantal's disappearance hadn't changed that much, though it had changed it some. Two shots of scotch was more than he used to drink in a week.

He finished his drink and the bartender, a man by the name of Buddy Wiser—who endured to no end the lamebrain jokes about his name—brought the bottle over and set it on the counter next to him. "Another?"

Will covered his glass.

"It's on the house."

"Thanks, but I'll pass." He got up, feeling a little lightheaded, though probably not so much by the scotch as by the fact that he hadn't moved from the bar for nearly three hours. "Think it's time I better get home."

One of the reasons he found himself at the Stop Over every night was because he didn't want to find himself at home. The house had grown into a mausoleum, a huge, vacuous space, void of everything beautiful and loving that had made up his life. Rachel was back with her parents. Not permanently, she had tried to assure him. Just until Chantal came back. Without Chantal, the house was simply too much to bear.

It was too much to bear for Will as well.

But he didn't have anywhere else to go.

He tucked in the tail of his shirt where it had pulled free, then zipped up his jacket and looked from the door to the bartender, wondering—like most of the people of Kingston Mills wondered these days—if he was going to make it all the way home tonight without becoming one of the missing.

"See you tomorrow," he said on his way out.

"I'll be here," Buddy answered.

Outside, Will stood on the sidewalk and gazed down the line of old mercury vapor lamps that cast a soft, ghostly glow over the empty street. There was a cool breeze out tonight. He could hear the rustle through the few remaining leaves on the maple trees in the park across the way. That was the only sound he could hear. The people of Kingston Mills did not stay out at night anymore. *No sense tempting the fates,* as Robert Underwood had put it.

No, no sense at all.

What happened next would never be completely

clear in his mind. All he remembered clearly was this: the night sky was all stars, the air was crisp, and he could see his own breath fog up in front of him as he stepped off the curb to cross the street. A cold front had swept down from Oregon the night before, dropping the temperature to an unseasonably twenty-six degrees. The thermometer had battled back to thirty-eight during the day, but when the sun had gone down, the temperature had plummeted again. The street was littered with patches of ice, many as black as the asphalt itself. Will remembered stepping around more than one. And he remembered seeing a car come around the corner in the distance, its headlights on high beam, nearly blinding him.

That's all he remembered, until he woke up in the hospital.

Rachel was standing over him, holding his hand. There were tears in her eyes, though she had managed to keep them from spilling over the rim. "Welcome back."

"Thanks," Will said through the fog. "Where have I been?"

"The Twilight Zone, I suspect."

He closed his eyes again. There was an incredible throbbing ache pounding away at the back of his head. It felt as if someone had cracked a baseball bat over his skull. "And where am I?"

"The hospital."

"How did I—?" He made a feeble attempt at sitting up, then fell back again.

"Take it easy, honey. You need to rest. The doctor said you gave the back of your head quite a whack."

"What happened?"

"Apparently, you slipped on a patch of ice." Rachel tried a smile, but behind the smile was the unmistakable presence of worry. "Oh, Will, I don't know what I would have done if I had lost you, too."

He squeezed her hand. "Hey, I'm still here, aren't I?"

"Yeah."

"So quit worrying, you're giving me a headache."

Her smile broadened. "Bet it hurts."

"Dreadfully. You can't imagine."

"The doctor says there's no fracture. So at least that's something. I think he was a little surprised by the X-rays. Especially after the way you looked when they brought you in."

"I guess it pays to have a hard head after all."

Rachel squeezed *his* hand this time, then sniffled and wiped away the rim of tears that still hadn't overflowed. She had always been a beautiful woman, from the very moment he had first bumped into her going into the old Cascade Theater in Redding. But she had never been quite as beautiful as she was at this moment, he thought.

"Things will be all right," he said.

"I know."

"It's been a nightmare lately . . ." He had intended to say something about what a screw-up he'd been the last six weeks, about how he was going to knock off the evening visits to the Stop Over, and about how—from this point on—he was going to do whatever it took to get Chantal back again. But something had caught his eye. Will sat up. "Do you see that?"

"What?"

He pointed to a place on the wall, below the clock, adjacent to the door. He wasn't positive, but he thought there had been some sort of chart hanging there a minute ago. The chart was gone now. In its place was a strange, watery opening, rectangular in shape, nearly as big as the doorway. As he stared at it, Will could see ripples forming across the black surface, like white caps, popping up, then disappearing again. "That!"

Rachel glanced at the wall, unimpressed. "The chart?"

"No, where the chart used to be."

She could have looked at him as if he were crazy and needed a little patronizing. *That* would have driven him crazy. But she didn't do that. She looked at the wall and then again at him. "The chart's right there, Will."

"You don't see that?"

"See what?"

"The opening in the wall? It's right there for God's sake!"

She checked again, bless her heart. But by the time she turned back to him, the opening had already begun to disintegrate. He watched the black, watery hole evaporate one droplet at a time as if it had been some sort of temporary aberration in the structure of the hospital. Only he thought it was more likely a temporary aberration somewhere inside his head.

A small patch of the wall appeared, peeking through the blackness in a splash of beige paint, first here, then there, until gradually he could see the chart that had been hanging below the clock. It was a life-size chart of the body's circulatory system. Near the heart, the last of the black, watery aberration glimmered, then vanished.

Will fell back against the pillow, meeting with a horrible shot of pain. He groaned.

"You hit your head pretty hard on the road base," Rachel said, moving up to the edge of being patronizing now. He might have even called her on it, but he *had* hit his head. And though she hadn't accused him yet, he wasn't so certain that he wasn't seeing things. "The doctor said it was a miracle you didn't crack your skull open."

"Yeah," he said lightly, "But you should have seen the pavement."

She smiled uneasily, and they shared a moment of silence that seemed as awkward as the first time he had worked up the nerve to kiss her. He had always believed that she had been embarrassed for him at that moment, and he believed now that she was embarrassed for him again. He had seen something that wasn't there.

Will looked past her at the chart on the wall. No black, watery hole. No opening to who knew where. No hint that anything else had ever hung there.

It hadn't really been there, had it?

That black, watery hole?

It had all been a figment of his imagination, a side effect of the concussion he must have endured when his head had struck the pavement.

Will wanted to believe that.

He wanted to believe it more than anything in the world.

Then why was it so hard?

VI

It was so hard because it hadn't been a figment of his imagination at all. Will Cassidy came to understand this explicitly over the next several weeks.

He was released from the hospital after a little more than thirty-six hours of bed rest and observation. There were still the occasional headaches, though they came less often now and they carried a far more tolerable bang. Besides, he could learn to handle the headaches. It was the black, watery holes that were giving him trouble.

He had detected two more of the aberrations. The first . . . in the hospital cafeteria while eating lunch. The hole appeared in the side of the serving counter and ran horizontal beneath the glass sneeze guard. Unlike the first one, this opening—all the while undulating—remained solid for nearly ten minutes as he sat there eating a salad and watching in utter fascination.

The second aberration was a beast of a different nature. He had been walking back to his room after a short tour of duty on the balcony, where for the first time in several days, he was able to breathe some fresh air and feel the warmth of the afternoon sun against his face. The hole appeared beneath a gurney sitting idly in the hallway outside one of the rooms. It was that same black, waterlike opening.

He had reasoned endlessly with himself about the holes, arguing on the one hand that they couldn't possibly exist or he wouldn't be the only person who could see them. On the other hand, since he *was* the only person who could see them, did that mean there was something wrong with him? That he might want to take a closer look at his personal mental hygiene, as he had heard it expressed on the radio once?

But this hole had been even stranger.

Something had poked its hand through the opening.

It was a moment of overwhelming, holy terror. The fear grabbed Will by the heart and shoved him up against the wall and held him there. He watched the fingers flex open, then writhe in the air as if they were trying to gauge the temperature. They were not normal fingers, normal in the sense of being flesh-toned. Instead, they had an eerie metallic, almost chromelike coloring. Four fingers and a thumb. Everything was there. But it wasn't human.

The hand extended out of the blackness, halfway up the forearm and wrapped its fingers around the edge of the gurney as if it were trying to pull itself free. It seemed to struggle there momentarily. And then another hand, fleshed in the same metallic coloring, emerged from the blackness only inches away. It was this second hand that seemed to sense the hole was going to close. It pulled back almost immediately, vanishing down into the nothingness.

Seconds later, the disintegration began. Millions of black particles began to break away from the hole and vanish, one after the other. It brought to mind a picture of raindrops rising back into the clouds to regroup again in some other place, at some other time.

The hand released its grip on the metal frame and disappeared into the blackness.

The last of the hole vanished.

The aluminum legs of the gurney came back into view, the beige wall followed.

Will released a breath that felt as if it had been burning a hole in his lungs. He slumped back against the wall, his hands on his knees, trying to calm himself. A cold sweat had broken out across his forehead. He wiped away the perspiration, still working at getting his breathing under control.

He had seen what he had seen, and now he knew—it was real.

Oh, God, it was real.

VII

He considered it, but in the end, Will decided not to say anything to Rachel. It was too easy to recall the look on her face in the hospital. She might not have felt sorry for him, but she *had* felt concerned. He had seen it in her face.

For a day or two after he returned home, she hovered over him, mothering him like she had when they had first started going together. It would have been better appreciated, he supposed, if he had been able to keep his mind off what had happened. But by the second day, he was growing more and more irritable, and Rachel began to pull back.

"What's gotten into you?" she asked him after he had snapped at her about leaving the dishes in the sink to soak. "Are you sure you're all right?"

"I'm fine. I'm just tired of seeing the dishes stack up."

"Then maybe you should think about washing them," she said, standing at the kitchen doorway. "I thought we agreed that Chantal came first over everything. That you and I were going to put all our efforts in getting her back . . . careers and housework be damned."

"We did."

"Then what the hell's this all about?"

It was about little black, watery holes that unfolded here and there and wherever in the fabric of space and time. It was about not being sure that when he closed the door if there was really a door there at all. It was about being . . . terrified.

"I don't know," Will said apologetically. "I guess I haven't been feeling quite right since the accident."

"You want me to call the doctor?"

The doctor had asked him to make a follow-up appointment in two weeks, just to make sure all the synapses inside his skull were still firing the way they were supposed to. Will, though, had no intentions of ever returning to that hospital again. Not if he had any say in the matter.

"No, I'll be all right."

VIII

Maybe eventually he might have been all right . . . if that had been the end of it. But the next day, while sitting in the den, he became aware of what appeared to be a hot spot forming in the bookcase across the room. It started out a soft, glowing red, the color of charcoal briquettes when they've finally started to produce some heat. The glow turned bright, then seemed to burn itself out, leaving in its wake the one thing Will was hoping he would never have to see again . . . another black, watery hole.

The opening grew to a span that ran from floor to ceiling, maybe three or four feet wide. A doorway of some sort, he speculated. Or a general fault in the operating system of reality. He wanted to laugh at that analogy, but couldn't bring himself to smile. Jesus, it was happening again. And this time, it was happening in his own house.

He didn't know how long the aberration—if he could still refer to it as such—held him there, frozen. But eventually he was able to stand up and push the chair away. He crossed the room, only distantly aware of the stiffness in his legs, and pulled a book down from the shelves. *Bartlett's Familiar Quotations,* a volume he sometimes used in his writings.

The blessing, he supposed, at least at this point, was that nothing had come clawing its way through. After that little episode with the hands at the hospital, he had spent endless hours wondering what lay on the other side. He had also wondered, though it had been brief and mostly ignored, if the holes were somehow related to all the recent disappearances.

He stood to one side, trying to peer into the glossy black vent and found it impossible to see beneath the watery surface. Exactly what the book was going to prove was anyone's guess, but as he stood there, he could feel a draft, slightly on the cool side, flowing silently through the opening. In his mind that proved one thing at the very least . . . a minimum of three dimensions were involved. The book was not going to bounce back.

Not unless someone—or some*thing*—threw it back.

It was a heavy volume, a hardback, five or six pounds if he had to guess. He stared down at it, then said a silent prayer. The worst scenario to scamper through his thoughts—his synapses were working quite well, the doctor would be pleased to hear—was this: just before the book arrived at its destination, a hand would reach out from the other side and catch it. That was not what happened, thank God.

He let the book sail and it was swallowed in one huge gulp.

Gone.

Just like that.

Not even a noticeable disturbance in the watery surface.

It was true then—this vent, or whatever you wanted to call it, was some sort of doorway between the here and now and . . .

And what? he wondered.

And whatever was on the other side.

Will leaned back against the window sill, his stomach clenched in a knot. He had been saving a place in his mind for a chance that the book might simply pass through the vent, bounce off the case behind it, and the aberration would vanish into a cartoonish puff of smoke. No such luck, though. This was the real thing.

What was *on the other side?* he wondered.

He had a caught a glimpse of it, he supposed.

Those metalliclike hands that had reached out of the blackness from beneath the gurney at the hospital, *they* were on the other side. And whatever they were attached to. But what else?

Just go ahead and do it before it's too late.

"Why not," Will whispered.

It didn't matter how close he stood, it was impossible to see past the black, watery surface. It was almost as if the liquidlike veil were there to form a seal of some sort. He touched it with the index finger of his right hand, immediately pulling the finger back. Not because he had encountered heat or cold—though it *was* slightly on the cool side—or even pain for that matter, but simply to make certain that if he was in danger of hurting himself it would be kept to a minimum.

The black, watery vent had swallowed the finger to the first knuckle, and the aberration had felt exactly the way it looked . . . as if it were formed of liquid. The interesting difference, however, was that it had left no residue on his skin. The finger had come back perfectly dry.

Will tried again. This time, he allowed not only his finger, but all of his right hand to dip into the liquid veneer. It felt as if he were dipping into a tub of thick shampoo, the viscous liquid closing in around his pores, sealing them from the surrounding air. He stretched his fingers, then closed them into a fist, taking a certain pleasure in the strange sensation.

It couldn't all be like this, could it?

There has to be something besides this damn liquid, doesn't there?

These thoughts crossed his mind almost simultaneously and were quickly followed by the realization that the vent was beginning to break up. Will pulled his hand free and fell back. The aberration's outer edges dissipated into the air, a thousand tiny dots at a time, like the dismantling of a giant jigsaw puzzle.

The cool draft fell still.

The last of the vent vanished.

Will, his back pushed up against the desk, stared at the bookcase with a mix of excitement and dread. There was a chance, he thought, his heart might actually explode from his chest cavity, it was pounding so savagely.

He raised his hand to the light.

Four fingers and a thumb.

Nothing out of the usual.

Thank God.

IX

That wasn't the last of it.

Less than a day later, it happened again.

He had gone into town to see the printer, who had been volunteering both his time and resources to printing posters of the missing Kingston Mills citizens. First, though, Will had needed to stop off to get a haircut, something he had overlooked for nearly six weeks now. He was only a block away from the Four Corners Barber Shop when a new vent opened in the display window of Mary Anne's Department Store across the street.

As Will had learned to do when he first spotted a vent, he stopped and checked the surroundings to see if anyone else had become aware of what was happening. Mrs. Schuster, who somctimes worked as a waitress at the Lakehead Inn, was crossing the middle of the street half a block up. Behind her, Terry Byrne and his five-year-old son, Andy, had stopped to window shop at the Book Mark. And there was a car Will didn't recognize, waiting at the stop light at Main and Pine. None of them appeared to be aware of what was going on.

Will stepped to the edge of the sidewalk, his hand wrapped absently around the pole of a street sign which limited parking to no longer than twenty minutes. Only distantly did he become aware of Mrs. Schuster as she reached the other side of the street and started up the sidewalk.

A hay devil—something you rarely saw this time of year in Kingston Mills—swept up several scraps of paper and carried them, swirling into the air in front of the woman. Mrs. Schuster swatted at a candy wrapper near her face, and then . . .

(just like that)

. . . it happened.

It happened so fast that at first Will found himself frozen in place, not sure he could even believe what his eyes had seen. What he had seen was this: as Mrs. Schuster went strolling past the vent, something had come out of the blackness and snatched her. Will wanted to believe that it was a man he had seen, but it was like no man he had ever seen before. He was maybe five feet tall, thin, wearing a lightweight jacket over a T-shirt, both the same color, which was not really a color at all. It was something metalliclike, almost chromelike, and even more surprising . . . it matched the man's pigmentation perfectly. There was one more thing. He was wearing goggles, slightly too big for his face, the frames and lenses shaded in that same metallic hue.

Mrs. Schuster's purse, which had slid off her arm, dropped to the ground with a thud and the surroundings immediately fell silent. Will glanced up the street at Terry Byrne and his son, who were still transfixed by whatever it was on display at the Book Mark. The car at the stop light had turned right and disappeared. No one else had seen what had happened.

Only Will.

He was the only one who could see the vents, the only one who could see what had just come out of the vents, the only one who knew what was happening to all the missing people.

The black, watery surface of the vent had rippled slightly as Mrs. Schuster had been pulled into it, but it was calm now as Will made his way across the street. He stepped onto the sidewalk, without having put what he was about to do into words yet. It was nothing more than a picture in his head, taken from somewhere far behind him.

He brushed his left shoulder against the light pole, took a few quick steps for momentum, and went sailing into the vent, hands out front, eyes closed, anybody's guess where he was going to end up. He did it all in a single movement, without a moment's hesitation, thinking only of Chantal. If he had thought of anything else, he wouldn't have been able to do it.

On the other side, he landed hard against a concrete walkway, rolled twicc, and jammed his shoulder into a bench that kept him from rolling into the street. The impact emptied his lungs in one, huge eruption of air. He grabbed for his midsection, fighting to get the breath back, his mouth working the air like a fish out of water. When it finally came, it burned a path down his windpipe and into his lungs. He gasped and sat back, grateful to be alive.

It was another thirty seconds before he was able to take in his surroundings with any measure of discerning. The black, watery surface of the vent where he had come through had settled again. Will made note of that before anything else, with a footnote to himself that at least temporarily he still had a way to get back. The strange thing was that he wasn't sure how far he had actually come.

He was lying on the sidewalk in front of Mary Anne's Department Store, almost as if he had bounced off the vent and had fallen to the ground. But he had gone through the vent; he was certain of that. And this wasn't Mary Anne's Department Store. At least it wasn't the one where Chantal had bought her first party dress for last year's Sadie Hawkins dance. It was close, the design, the items in the window, the name, its location on the street. Close. But the store was like everything else here: it had no color. Like the sidewalk beneath him, the bench he had rolled into, the streets, the other buildings, like all of it . . . it was a blinding, crippling monochrome.

Same as the man, Will thought.

Out of the corner of his eye, he caught a movement

and tried to pull his feet, which were splayed across the sidewalk, back into his body. It was a boy he had seen, maybe a year or two younger than Chantal. In his hands, he held a comic book, the lettering and illustrations all done in a strange sort of three-dimensional embossing.

That's how they work around the monochrome, Will thought distantly.

He had pulled his feet back, but he had not pulled them back far enough to prevent the boy from tripping over them. It wasn't a bad stumble, just a missed step or two before the boy caught his feet again. Then there was a moment when the boy looked down at Will with annoyance, and Will realized it was the kind of annoyance you shoot at a high spot in the sidewalk. As if the boy had not actually seen him there at all, but had looked right through him.

"Sorry," Will said, startled by the sound of the word as it came out of his mouth. It had sounded amplified somehow, and drawn out, almost guttural. This place was not only different by its lack of color, he realized, but also by the distortion of its sounds.

The boy disappeared down the street.

Heading for the Collector's Corner, Will thought as he climbed to his feet. He brushed the monochrome dust off his jacket sleeves and the front of his pants, then looked up the street, past the five-and-dime at the bookstore (which was called the Book Cover on this side). Beyond the bookstore, he could see the sign for the barbershop, and beyond that, in the distance, just a glimpse of Hattie's Antiques.

Where to start?

The Abductor (as Will had already come to think of him) had taken Mrs. Schuster somewhere nearby. It couldn't have been far, because Will had come through the vent only seconds later. How far could they have gotten in a matter of seconds?

Only two places came to mind. The first was an old warehouse that had been split into a machine shop on one side and a wrecking yard on the other. That place was right around the corner, less than two blocks from here. The other place was the old abandoned railroad station, up the street and to the left. The kids liked to play there. At least they did on the Kingston Mills side. Then there was a third possibility, now that he thought about it—the Haberstock Mill, which had been closed down in the late sixties. It sat near the edge of town, though, a fairly decent hike from here.

It was the warehouse, then.

That's where he would start.

X

It was surprising how disorienting the monochromed landscape could be. As he moved down the street, he found it next to impossible to simply put one foot in front of the other without weaving unsteadily. Everything felt slightly off center.

He managed to stay on his feet, though, at least long enough to make it to the old warehouse. The machine shop, a place called Anderson's Tool and

Die, was closed on Sundays, according to a sign posted in the window next to the door. Will leaned against the glass, his hands cupped around his eyes, and tried to get a peek inside, but it was too dark to see anything.

Next door, there was a man out front dismantling what looked like an old Ford Pinto. He had just ignited a cutting torch and had flipped the visor to his helmet when Will walked past him.

Otto's Auto Wrecking was the name of the place. It was not a far cry from the junk yard that sat in the same spot on the pigmented side of Kingston Mills. The same corrugated tin panels (only monochromed, of course). The same caustic mix of oil and gasoline in the air. And while Will had only been there once or twice, he had learned that the only way to find what you were looking for was to start scavenging through the piles one by one. This time, though, he was scavenging for something a little different.

He checked the office first, then a small machine shop in the back, another room that appeared to be used for warehousing small parts, and finally a bathroom where the monochromed dirt, several shades darker, was visibly noticeable. Chantal was nowhere to be found. Neither were any of the other missing Mills residents.

On his way out, it occurred to him that if no one could see him, then he must be to this world what the Abductor was to the colorized version of the Mills . . . some sort of invisible predator. He didn't know how he felt about that, but he couldn't imagine feeling good.

At the curb, he stopped to get his bearings and was surprised to discover that a new vent had opened across the street. It consisted of that same black, watery surface, about the size of a doorway, this one overlying the front of a brick building. It had not been there when he had entered the wrecking yard.

He stepped forward, curious. There were the usual questions that came to mind about how long it might remain open. But the question that was most unsettling was this: Did this mean the other vent had closed and he wouldn't be able to get back again?

Before he could give it much thought one way or the other, the vent began to disintegrate. In a matter of seconds, it had splintered into millions of minute particles, each particle evaporating almost as quickly as it had been formed.

The vent disappeared.

Will sank back against a light pole.

Somewhere inside him it felt as if a hole had opened and it was slowly devouring any hope he might have of ever finding Chantal again. He felt that and he felt something else. He felt a strange weariness working its way into his bones like a strain of super flu. It hadn't hit him yet, not fully at least, but it was—

Half a block up, the Abductor came running around the corner. He was wearing his goggles—the monochromed version of sunglasses, Will imagined—and carrying a small rectangular box in his hands. No sooner was he around the corner, than he glanced down at the box and suddenly dropped out of his sprint. He walked a few steps further, then came to a standstill, visibly disappointed.

Too late, Will thought. *The vent's already closed. That's what that little box of yours just told you, isn't it?*

The Abductor turned around, his shoulders slumped, and headed back the way he had come.

Will took after him.

XI

They ended up not at the old railroad station or the Haberstock Mill as Will had originally thought they might, but at a private residence one block over from the city park. On the colorized side of Kingston Mills, this was a house that used to be occupied by Henry Bascom and his wife, Edith. They had packed up and moved south to the Bay Area after the mill had shut down. To the best of Will's knowledge no one had occupied the place since. That was on the colorized side.

On this side, things were apparently a little different.

The Abductor climbed the front steps of the old Victorian and entered the house, stopping only a moment to check the box in his hands one last time. Will went through a side gate to the back of the house. In the far back corner, at the end of the gravel driveway, sat an old detached garage. He peered through the window at the darkened interior, looking past the car (which resembled a Plymouth Duster), and finding nothing much else of interest.

The house, assuming the layout didn't stray far from the Bascom house's, was a beautiful two-story Victorian with three bedrooms and a bath upstairs;

the living room, a parlor, a kitchen, and a huge walk-in pantry downstairs. There was also an attic and a basement.

Will leaned against the corner of the garage, feeling slightly short of breath and wondering what was wrong with him. Through the back-porch windows, he watched the Abductor fiddle around in the kitchen, then disappear back into the depths of the house. A moment later, the light in the basement went on.

That's where you've got 'em, isn't it, you crazy bastard?

Two short casement windows had been mounted just above ground level on either side of the back porch. Will got down on his knees, then his stomach and peered into the basement. He would never admit to being surprised, because surprise was only the tip of the iceberg. They were all there: Elmo Stanton. Chantal. Mrs. Schuster. All of them. The Abductor had them sealed off in a corner of the room, caged liked animals. But at least they were there and they were alive.

The casement windows were locked. He looked around for something he could use to break them open, and when he found nothing, he took a more direct approach. He sat back and landed a solid right shoe to the centerpiece of the sash. The frame collapsed into the room, followed almost immediately by both panes of glass.

Will went through, driven more by adrenaline than thought.

The Abductor, who had been toying with the rectangular box at his work bench, turned, the startle unmistakable. The box slipped out of his hands and landed on the concrete floor, somehow remaining intact. One hand shot up to cover his eyes, while the other grabbed for the goggles, which were hanging around his neck. He worked them into place, then seemed to gain control of himself again. He smiled sardonically.

"Out of your element?" he asked. His speech was marked by that same dronelike, low-pitched slur that seemed to mark all the sounds in this place.

"You're the one wearing the goggles."

"Minor inconvenience. Temporary. Until I adapt." He was a nervous little man, full of high energy, rocking from foot to foot. It was hard to imagine him ever relaxing, ever closing his eyes and sleeping.

"Adapt?" Will asked.

"To your side. Yes."

"Then the vents that keeping popping everywhere, they're . . . yours?"

"Apertures. Yes. Mine." He smiled, almost to himself. "There's here . . . and then there. All bright sights and clear sounds. You don't appreciate it. Yes. Can't appreciate it. No."

Behind him, someone stirred. Will didn't turn to see who it was because he didn't want to take his eyes off the Abductor. Not for a second. But when he heard the voice, even in that low-pitched slur, he knew immediately that it was Chantal.

"Daddy, you're here. How did you get here?"

"Are you all right?"

"I'm just a little tired, that's all."

The Abductor grinned at him. "Tired? You, too? Yes?"

He *was* feeling tired. Not sleepy tired, but worn-out

tired. And it was something he preferred to keep to himsclf. "Tell me . . . why all the people?"

"Think of your bodies, then of mine. Think of physiology. Yes?"

It made perfect sense once he thought about it. Chantal and the others . . . they were test subjects, guinea pigs, a means of understanding how the body handles all the sounds and colors. The stimuli was like a narcotic to him. There was the pleasurable experience, and then there was the overload. He was trying to master the overload.

"This is all on your own, isn't it?" Will asked quietly.

"Of course. Who else?"

"No one else even knows what you're doing here."

"No one."

Will glanced back at Chantal, who was standing now, with her hands wrapped around the monochromed bars. Her face was drawn, deep lines that didn't belong there etched into her cheeks, shadows beneath her eyes. He didn't want to stretch this out any longer than necessary.

"It's time to let them go," he said calmly. "They have families and—"

"No. They stay."

Then someone from behind him said, "He keeps the key in the drawer there, under the work bench."

Will made the mistake of turning to see who was talking—it was Elmo Stanton. In that instant, the Abductor closed the distance between them and struck Will hard across the side of the face with something that felt like a baseball bat. Will fell back against the door to the cage, hitting his head against the metal bars, and thinking distantly to himself that he knew better than to take his eyes off this guy. How could he have been so stupid?

Somewhere far away, he heard Chantal scream, "Daddy!"

The Abductor closed again, and Will could see this time that it wasn't a baseball bat he was holding in his hands. It was a gardening hoe. He swung it again and it landed near the crown of Will's head, leaving behind a strange numbness that seemed less painful than disorienting. Will backed into the bars and curled up.

It shouldn't hurt this bad, he thought from faraway.

"Not so big on this side. Not so strong," the Abductor said.

"Stop it!" Chantal screamed. "You're hurting him!"

The Abductor reached back for another swing, and this time Will was able to get his arm up to block it. The handle of the hoe landed flush across his fore-arm. It hurt, there was no mistaking the hurt, but he was still able to grab on.

"Let go! Let go!"

He didn't have the strength to wrestle the hoe away, but he managed to hook his arm over the handle and lock the blade behind him. With a violent tug, the Abductor dragged Will across the concrete floor, away from the cage, as if he were nothing more than a house dog with his teeth clenched around one end of an old rag.

"Not strong here. Just a tired old man. Yes."

It was true. Will hated to admit it to himself, but it

was true. For whatever the reason, every movement he made seemed to drain his strength a little more. This little, five-foot troll was going to overpower him, and there wasn't much he was going to be able do about it.

The Abductor dragged him another couple of feet across the floor, Will holding on for dear life, and then he stopped and bent over in another attempt to wrestle the hoe from Will's grasp. Instinctively, Will fumbled for something to grab onto—a hand, an arm, a fistful of hair, anything. What he came up with were the goggles.

The Abductor let out an immediate scream that sounded like pure agony. He dropped the hoe and fell back, shading his eyes with his hands. For a moment, as he was stooped over and trying to rub the pain out of his eyes, he resembled the Hunchback of Notre Dame—a sad, almost sympathetic, little man.

Will climbed to his feet, sucking air and feeling like a man twice his age. It was all he could do just to toss the hoe aside and pick up the goggles.

"The keys!" someone yelled from behind him.

He found them in the drawer, where Elmo had said they would be, and tossed them to Chantal, who unlocked the cell. "Why don't you take everyone upstairs," he said. "And wait for me out front. All right?"

"What are you going to do?"

"Just say good-bye, that's all."

The Abductor, who had huddled into the far corner with his hands still covering his eyes, peeked through the thin splay of fingers like a child checking to see if the monster was still there. "Can't go," he said. "No."

Will crossed the room and picked up the rectangular box that had earlier been dropped. It was what he had expected—some sort of electronic grid, all done in monochrome and three dimensions, similar to a relief map. He ran his fingers over the surface, trying to decipher the landmarks, and suddenly the box began to put out a low-pitched vibration. A moment later, a small square, enclosing an X, rose up out of the grid in what could only be construed as some sort of electronic marker.

"I do believe you've got another vent opening up," he said. He thought their current location was landmarked by a circle within a circle, which meant the vent wasn't more than a block or two away. "Guess it's time for me to be getting back home. I appreciate the map."

"No. Leave the map." The Abductor made a feeble attempt to reach out and grab him with one hand.

Will pushed him away with almost no effort, which was a good thing, because he didn't have much effort left. The fatigue wasn't getting any worse, but it wasn't getting any better, either. "Sorry. No can do."

"Please!"

"Maybe next time." On his way out, Will stopped at the top of the stairs and looked back. The Abductor had crossed the room and was standing at the bottom, looking up through splayed fingers, still cringing from the blinding colors.

He isn't going to give up, Will thought. *This is all he has, all he is.*

Out front, he met up with the group again. Lily Hanover was leaning against a four-by-four porch support, looking as tired as he had ever seen her. "Don't you hate it?" she said.

"What?"

"Everything painted this silvery metallic color. No blues or yellows or reds. No rainbows. No flat white. No glossy black. It's enough to drive a person insane, don't you think?"

Will nodded and looked down at the map in his hands. He didn't think the new vent could be far from here, and when he glanced up to gain his bearings, it was a pleasant surprise to find it across the street, only two houses down.

Chantal came up beside him and put her arm around his waist. "How do we get out of here?"

"Right there," he said, pointing at the vent. Only she wouldn't be able to see it; he had forgotten that little fact. If he hadn't fallen and struck his head, he wouldn't have been able to see it, either. "Come on, I'll show you."

They crossed the street as a group, moved down the sidewalk, and came to a stop in front of a rundown Victorian that Charlie Weaver had inherited from his father two years ago. He hadn't got around to renovating the house yet, but it was something he said he had always wanted to do. The vent was at the foot of the front porch steps, shimmering black, open for now, but for how long no one knew.

Will stepped up next to it. "Elmo, why don't you come on up here. You were the first one to have to endure this nightmare. Let's see if we can't get you home again."

"What the hell you talking about, Will Cassidy?"

"Just trust me, all right?"

Elmo stepped forward. Will took him by the arm and guided him up the first step and through the vent. He crossed over one piece at a time, with his right leg disappearing first, followed shortly by his left arm. In less than a breath, the black, watery vent had closed in around him and he was gone.

Bobby Cutler came up and stood next to Will. "Where'd he go?"

"Home. He went home, Bobby."

"Can I go next?"

"Sure." He ushered the boy up to the steps, his hand resting in the small of Bobby's back. "All you have to do is climb the steps."

"That's it?"

"That's it."

"Will I see you on the other side?"

"In a few minutes. Now, go on."

After Bobby, Lily Hanover went next, and then Teresa Saunders and Mrs. Schuster, until one by one they had all stepped through the vent—Chantal being the last—and Will was the only one left behind. He glanced down the street, then down at the grid map in his hand. The emblem for the vent—the square with the X in its center—had begun to vibrate again. That could only mean one thing. The vent was getting ready to close.

Chantal called out from the other side. "Daddy?"

"I'm coming, baby." He took the first step up, then the second, and suddenly found himself straddling the two worlds, caught half-here and half-there. Something had caught him from behind. When he turned and stuck his head back through the vent, he discovered that the Abductor had taken hold of the tail of his jacket. The little man was tugging for all he was worth.

Chantal, who was standing at the foot of the steps in front of him, reached out for his hand. "What's wrong?"

"He's got hold of my jacket," Will said, acutely aware that the outer edges of the vent had begun to break into thousands of tiny, swarming specs. In a matter of seconds, they were going to start flying off, tens of thousands at a time, and he didn't want to know what that would do to him. "You've gotta help me through!"

"Someone help!" Chantal screamed. "He's caught!"

Adam Walker, a man Will had never met before that day, came running up the walkway from the street, as did David Winters and Emily Sanders. Chantal motioned to Walker, the closest body. "Grab his hand!"

He grabbed Will around the wrist, using both hands, and together with Chantal, neither of them actually able to see the vent, they managed to pull him free. Or at least free of the vent. The Abductor was still holding on, half-in, half-out of the opening, his eyes clamped shut to the sudden brightness.

"No! You stay!" he was screaming.

It was too late to shed the jacket.

Too late to pry his hands loose.

The vent completed its disintegration in a matter of milliseconds.

Whoosh! It was gone.

The Abductor let out an agonizing scream.

His upper torso, from just above the shirt line, separated from the rest of him and fell to the ground in a lifeless heap. What remained behind was anyone's guess. It had either disintegrated with the vent, or it was lying on the ground in a similar heap on the other side. Either way, what was left here was a horrific mess.

For a long while, Will found himself holding Chantal against his chest, trying to spare her the gruesome sight. It was only later that he realized she couldn't have seen it anyway.

XII

Will doesn't talk about it anymore, but he worries sometimes.

The vents have never stopped opening and closing. They still pop up out of nowhere every once in awhile, and Will is still the only person who can see them.

And while no one else besides the Abductor has ever come through, he dreads the thought that someday that might change.

FUEL

Adam-Troy Castro

HE PENCILED THE WORDS ON AN ORDINARY THREE-BY-five index card, in scrupulously neat handwriting that respected the authority of parallel blue lines. Beneath the words he signed and printed his name, Gordon Wilson, then beneath that his street address, city, state, zip, and (with conscious absurdity) his phone number, all in writing remarkable for its evenly spaced precision, and for its utter absence of emotion, as if he were filling out a form for a magazine subscription and not an explanation for the bullet that he was about to fire through his brain. The note itself was a carefully thought-out compromise between explaining too much and not explaining enough, expressing all of his weariness and despair without ever going over the line into maudlin obviousness; he'd written notes much like it a dozen previous times in his life, always devoting so much time and effort to the perfect phrasing that he finally lost all heart for the actual act. But this time he had the words and the sentiment down cold, with the kind of inspired brevity that left nothing else to say.

The card read:

> *After all the hope, all the fear, all the self-hatred and all the futile lies spoken to myself in the middle of the night, I can finally admit I'm not getting better, I'm getting worse.*

He could have spent hours going into specifics: the anhedonia, the mood swings, the shattered friendships, the money problems, the loneliness, the failures, the hopelessness of a life where even managing to endure meant another day of watching the world crumble deeper into hell. But by the time he'd written all of that he would have lost the will—keeping the desire, and the increased self-loathing that always came with such broken promises.

He spent all that day in a state approaching peace, boarding his cats, vacuuming his apartment, paying off the last of his monthly bills, washing the car, then driving to a deserted parking lot behind an office supply warehouse that was never open on Tuesdays. Then he placed the card message side up on the dashboard, and he took precisely four deep breaths, and with absolutely no compunction at all placed the barrel between the lips and blew everything he was out the back of his head.

Despite all the advance publicity, he saw the bright light a fraction of a second *before* he died.

He did not have the time to realize how wrong that was, or to wonder why he should be afraid.

The Travelers lived in a gossamer place of juggling possibilities and oscillating time: a place that in all its particulars defied the laws of the greater universe outside, and therefore could be fairly considered a separate universe itself.

Their universe was a vehicle, designed to travel faster and farther than anything bound by mundane physics, and while its ultimate destination was far beyond the material world of planets and stars and solar systems, it did frequently slow down whenever it passed such places, to collect its equivalent of fuel.

Fuel:

Chitinous crablike thing, dragging itself painfully across semimolten rock, toward the sulphurous pool that will cause it to expire in agony.

Fuel:

Pulsating ball of sentient energy, once as bright as the stars, now so dim it barely qualifies as a spark, eschewing the flammable breezes that would fully ignite it again.

Fuel:

Dark shambling predator, all teeth and hunger, despondent for lack of anything else to kill, standing at the edge of a howling maelstrom, and gathering enough will to hurl itself in.

Fuel:

Floating bag of hydrogen, bobbing to and fro in a wind-tossed upper atmosphere, sinking deeper and deeper into the darkness as it consciously refrains from the chemical processes that keep it bouyant and aloft and alive.

Fuel:

Unknown failure of a man, swallowing the barrel of a revolver as he imagines this the moment of his release: taking comfort in the thought that the thought he thinks now is the last thought he'll think forever.

Fuel:

Unknown thousands of others.

Creatures who once inhabited worlds from across the entire breadth of time and space, each one a fugitive from a life so different from all the others that to them its most primitive thought would be a code unbreakable, in a tongue alien and unspoken.

Each one despairing. Each one urging itself toward death.

Each one captured in the net.

Added to the mix.

Burning, among the fuel.

For Gordon Wilson, the first moment of his new existence was a headlong plunge into Hades.

None of what he saw or heard or tasted or smelled had any direct analogue to human experience. But he had been a human being, with a mind formed by his human life; and even as he plummeted past the bright light into a place he could only comprehend as darkness, he could only think that this was his punishment.

He hadn't expected to be punished; like almost all suicides, he'd expected not quite oblivion but the satisfaction of knowing that all his pain had ended. He had not expected to arrive in this strange place, surrounded by uncounted thousands of jabbering alien voices, all of whom seemed as horrified and repulsed by him as he was by them. He hadn't expected the sensation of being tapped, of being drained, of having everything he was wrung from his soul like washwater being wrung from a cloth. He hadn't expect the sheer vertigo of feeling his every memory played back, at impossible speed.

He hadn't expected to be fuel.

And that wasn't even the bad news . . .

The Travelers had had a mission, initially; one that had seemed simple enough to the creatures they had been. It had something to do with a crease through the process of entropy, and the swirling contradiction that was the passage of time. It had to do with the existence of a universe that refused to abide by the aesthetic laws of the thirteen major interdimensional constants, and the need to maintain strategic superiority in the places that probability had abandoned. All of this had seemed so obvious and vital once. But they'd changed, in the timeless time since putting their vessel together; some might even say, they'd degenerated. They were no longer the beings who'd set themselves an impossible task and built themselves a miraculous vessel to help them accomplish it; in that time they'd forgotten all of their arcane and hard-won knowledge and become passengers instead of engineers. Now the bubble piloted itself, without their input; and the glorious mission that had once been the whole reason for their existence now seemed nothing but an ancient folly, too far gone to change.

They wouldn't have understood Vietnam, but they would have sympathized.

They did not notice when the Fuel Acquisition mechanism picked up Gordon Wilson; since the process was automatic, and none of them were involved. They didn't notice when the entire vessel bucked and lurched in protest; since their living space was buffered, and did not stir at all even when subjected to turbulence that briefly threatened to tear their entire private universe apart. They did not feel even a moment of fear; they felt nothing, and were perfectly content with feeling nothing, even though they'd just revived something very ancient and very dangerous. They didn't have the slightest idea that anything was wrong, and they might not have cared even if somebody had come around to tell them.

In short, they were like the complacent everywhere in that they were already dead, and did not yet happen to know it . . .

Gordon Wilson first heard the distant laughter while he still believed himself a fresh inmate in the underworld. It wasn't laughter, really—there was no genuine sound in this place. But his mind still insisted on interpreting everything in human terms, and even as he reeled in a sea of alien images—

(rooted in sea bottom feeding on dregs, drifting through digestive tract absorbing random proteins, slogging through the lake of fire, gliding on the methane winds, colors not in any human spectrum, sins not in any human bible, thoughts not in any human lexicon, a billion separate forms of life, a billion separate ways to die, mother as great bloated sac filled with seeds, father as creature infected by parasite, children as playthings and as food, right-angles perceived as circles, abstractions perceived as shapes, viruses perceived as politics, death perceived as sustenance, despair perceived as fuel)

—Even as Gordon Wilson fought to preserve his sanity against a tidal wave of such mutually contradictory images, he heard the laughter building behind it all.

And he felt everything he'd ever been run cold with fear.

Because while he did not yet understand why . . . he recognized that laughter.

He recognized it in ways that went beyond memory, went beyond instinct. He recognized it in a manner that acknowledged he'd never personally heard it before. He recognized it in the manner of a man recognizing a sound that no man had ever heard, for as long as there had ever been men; which yet remained a sound that all men knew, since awareness of that sound was wired in the very genetic material that made them human. It was the sound of an ancient, immortal enemy, older than the world—an enemy whose own last moments before being imprisoned in this place were now played out for Gordon Wilson, at a volume that drowned out all else.

The Hunter stood beneath the night sky and stared up

at the lights as they receded, knowing that they meant his failure. There were thousands of them, more numerous than the stars; and they were all moving away so quickly that even his lightning-fast reflexes could not move his eyes fast enough to track them. The lights had taken him by surprise—he'd been advancing on the last settlement, and had eagerly anticipated killing all the remaining population by morning—but the instant he saw them, he knew that the hated ones had escaped, after all; despite lifetimes spent pursuing them from world to world, laying waste to all their defenses, leveling their cities, finding their bolt-holes, flushing them out and exterminating them, to the point where the last handful he was about to kill tonight were the very last to live and breathe anywhere in a universe that would have been purer and cleaner for their absence, they'd escaped. Oh, he could track the lights receding in the sky, for some idea which way they'd gone; but there were so many lights that the vast majority must have been unpiloted decoys, fired off into places where the hated ones had no intention of going. By the time he investigated even a few of the flight patterns, the creatures he'd spent his entire existence killing would have been well beyond his reach; though they themselves were dying, from all the plagues he'd sowed, they would still have more than enough time to travel beyond his reach, find some lifeless world, and infect it with their seed.

He'd been their greatest enemy, the one who went on hunting and chasing and killing and destroying, despite anything they could do to stop him. He'd reduced them from a cancer, metastasizing throughout the stars, to a terrified little community of defeated fugitives, who had to watch themselves wither and die while waiting for him to descend and erase their blot forever.

He'd never rested.

He'd never shown a moment's mercy.

He'd never lost a single battle.

He'd doomed even those who fled.

And it hadn't stopped them from winning.

The Hunter stood beneath the night sky, watching the stars spell out his defeat on a slate as large as the universe. And he did something that would have astonished those who for so long had considered him a soulless omnipotent destroyer—he wept, out of humiliation. He wept in the manner of any being whose life becomes an empty thing, without purpose or hope, who realizes that his entire existence has been for nothing, and that he has pitifully wasted every moment he stood alive beneath the stars. And then he succumbed to despair and he opened his veins and spilled out the last of his existence onto the dirt of the place that should have seen the culmination of all his dreams.

He, too, saw the bright light an instant before he died.

As he was captured in the net.

Added to the mix.

Set to burning, among the fuel.

And though the Hunter had spent the eons that followed content to be damned to the purgatory he felt he deserved, a merciful universe had just placed one of his enemy's descendants back within his reach . . . giving him a purpose again, for the first time in an interval longer than the lifetime of worlds. His despair was transformed into triumph, and he laughed. . . .

While Gordon Wilson, quailing, realized that there are some things worse than being joyless and afraid.

There was never any shortage of fuel because there was never any shortage of despair; it had always been far more common than hope, and there was always more being manufactured. But despair was a volatile fuel, that always needed to be stirred just right; unless properly refined, it transformed into hope or love or faith or hate or rage, which could be just as powerful but were even readier to change states without any prior warning. But that's why the Collectors were designed to gather fuel that wouldn't interact with the rest of the mix in any undesirable manner; any uncontrollable chemistry between one element and another could be, quite literally, explosive.

There had always been impurities. But they had always been dealt with, by automatic systems. Up until now, the catastrophic had been avoided.

But nobody could have predicted the sudden reunion between ancient Hunter and Ancient Prey.

Now, all of sudden, there was laughter polluting the mix. Cruel and hungry laughter, from the remains of he who'd stalked and killed; anticipatory laughter, from he who looked forward to the stalking and killing yet to come; joyful laughter, from he who'd felt no joy for eons. It was laughter with a voice, and that voice said, *After all these years you've come back to me! Giving me something to kill again,* and the maliciousness in its tone was so great that of the thousands of other creatures whose last moments had been rendered fuel, at least half were now contaminated by spasms of sympathetic fear.

The bubble lurched. Slowed. Went violently off-course and devastated a world of singing sentient oceans by instantly boiling them into dead clouds of superheated steam. The Travelers, secure in their cushioned habitat, didn't notice, and probably wouldn't have cared if they had. After all, they would have reasoned, wasn't their vessel nearly indestructible? Wasn't it designed to survive a whole lot worse than that?

And they would have had a point, more or less.

But the chain reaction had already begun.

Gordon Wilson stood paralyzed at the bottom of a well of madness, inundated by moments from the lives of creatures unimagined, hearing nothing but that hated laugh echoing in the darkness, seeing nothing but that hated shape which eclipsed all else as it drew toward him. He stood bound by all the failures of his life, all the ways in which he'd fallen short of being bold or smart or brave or enough, and he faced a thing that dwarved all men, that had been man's enemy for much longer than there'd been men to hate . . . and he knew there was no hope of escape, no hope of defiance, no hope of survival, no hope of anything but the inevitability of dying again.

And he felt an emotion as alien to him as any of those that pummeled him in the darkness: rage.

It's funny, isn't it?

After all, isn't this what they prepare us for all our lives?

When you're a child, and your mommy and daddy beat you for saying no, for fighting back, for seeing through their lies, for seeing them as the bullies they are, for refusing to make yourself as small as they want you to be? Don't they say, That's enough out of you! That's all I want to hear from you! Don't talk back! Now sit there and take your punishment until you apologize!

When you're in the playground, and the big kid sits on your chest and rubs the dirt on your face, and you squirm beneath his weight, loathing him, wanting him dead, knowing yourself powerless but vowing that he'll never make you cry, crying anyway because you're not great enough to contain all the pain and hate and humiliation? Don't they say, You brought this on yourself? You let him tease you? You showed him it bothered you and made yourself the victim?

When you sit at your desk in a plain white office even as the sky outside your window dims from blue to black, and your head turns to fog and your heart turns to stone and you look at the clock and you think of another day's long downward slide to death? And you know that there should be something more to life than this, that there should be some source of joy and hope and a reason for wanting to get up in the morning? And they say, Don't let it get you down, it's just your job, you may hate it and you may feel it sucking out your life but you can't just throw it away because you need to contribute, to pay the bills, to do what they tell you to do, and do it without protest because there's no escape from it anyway?

When you stand in the center of a busy city street surrounded by thousands of people all of whom seem better smarter prettier thinner happier and more fulfilled than you, and all the world seems a place that's left you out, that's locked you outside, that's deliberately left you uninvited, and you want to scream, Look at me, look at me, I'm here, I matter, I hurt, I need? And you do nothing because you know what they'd say if you did, which is that you're crazy, you're worthless, you're not worth the attention? And so you turn your face into a mask and you say nothing and you go with the flow and you turn all your anger and resentment into yet another dagger in your heart?

Isn't it all just the same message, endlessly repeated? Don't stand up. Don't fight back. Don't open your mouth. Don't walk on eggs. Don't take chances. Don't do anything but take what they give you.

Some of us don't listen. I did. It made me a rabbit, caught in the headlights. A pathetic little man, defeated without ever stirring himself to fight.

But then I never knew who the real enemy was. I never knew that all our history, all our wars, all our witch-hunts, all our genocides, all our rapes, all our crimes, all our murders, all our atrocities, all our lynchings, all our tyrannies, all our nightmares, all our Hell-legends, all our bogeymen, all our gods of evil, all the times we feared strangers in dark places, all the times we bubbled over with cruelty, all our weakness and all our cowardice and all our evil—that was just the part of us that remembered the past, and remained so afraid of being hunted down again that we searched for you in every unfamiliar face.

But this time I know who you are, and this time I have nowhere left to hide.

Come for me this time, you murdering bastard, and you're going down.

The bubble was supposed to be invisible and immaterial; it was supposed to journey beyond the places inhabited by mere things. It wasn't supposed to fade into existence any more frequently than it had to in order to collect its fuel.

But the fuel was changing composition, and the ride was getting bumpy.

The bubble appeared on a planet of mile-high volcanic spires, crashing across an entire hemisphere in an instant, scattering the pillars of stone like dominoes before once again fading away.

It appeared on a world of lush verdant jungle, skimming the forest canopy like a stone skimming the surface of a pond, and everywhere it touched the greenery withered, and the animals died, and the ground turned deadly and black.

It appeared within a sun that nurtured a world that was home to beings whose basest thoughts were the most brilliant poetry ever known; and in the instant it lingered there before moving on, the sun was reduced to a cinder, and the world to a mortuary.

It appeared in the midst of beings who were more gods than men, who had been fighting a war since the beginning of time; and it spun in their midst long enough to fatally distract one side and give the critical advantage to the other.

Completely out of control now, it described a completely random path through the universe, damaging or destroying a hundred different worlds with every instant; and somewhere along the way the life-support failed and the Travelers died in a burst of shock and incomprehension, but they were irrelevant. Because the chain-reaction was not over with, yet . . .

Deep inside, the essence of the Hunter went after the essence of essence of Gordon Wilson.

He came in the way that a crumbling mountain comes. He engulfed everything that lay in his path, swelling with rage and power with every moment, becoming even more fearsome than he had been in life. He was black and malicious and infinite and greater than any man's ability to comprehend him, and as he drew close to Gordon Wilson the mix bubbled with all the flavors of alien fear.

Gordon Wilson thought only of the blue windbreaker he owned in third grade.

It was a shiny blue jacket, of the sort that mothers find cute and kids find mortifying; Gordon had owned it for about six months. He'd hated it with a passion for several weeks after he first got it, not because of the way it looked during the day, but because of what it turned into at night: hanging on its hook on the back of his bedroom door, it became an apelike beast, with long clutching arms. It wasn't a fear that ruled him; even as he lay in bed, waiting for the beast to pounce, waiting for it to leap off his bedroom door and scrabble at his neck, he'd known perfectly well that it was just a jacket, rendered false and menacing by shadows. It should have been way too silly to worry about for even a moment. And yet even if he put the jacket in a closet or drawer, or left it downstairs, the knowledge that it was still out there, in the darkness, taking on the shape that it only took at night, had given him the sweats. It passed, of course. Time moved on, and with it came more sensible things to get frightened about. But Gordon had never forgotten the nights he'd spent afraid of that jacket, and the way he'd so briefly seen in its emptily hanging folds the shape of things to dread. He'd always wondered where such a crazy fear could have come from. Now he knew.

All around them, alien voices gibbered in confusion and fear. Gordon heard the cries of things that flew, the bubbling of things that swam, the soft hiss of things that crawled, the indescribable sound of things that had lived in manners beyond his comprehension. Whatever they were, wherever they'd come from, they'd all come to a point in their lives where life itself had seemed too much to ask of them. And though they'd wallowed in their despair ever since, they sensed what was happening in their midst, and were now afraid.

The essence of something that had possessed light gossamer wings flew at the Hunter, to stop him. Its thoughts were agony in color: dark purple starbusts, with pulsating emerald stripes. It was willing to give up anything in order to stop the Hunter. The Hunter batted it aside with the slightest twitch, leaving the mix black from its death throes.

The essence of something that had been a predator itself, that had lived to tear flesh from captive throats and then swallow the blood that came spurting from the wounds, pounced next. Its thoughts were the taste of salt and the odor of putrefaction. But it, too, was determined to protect Gordon Wilson from the

Hunter. It failed. The Hunter became two rows of glistening fangs that rent the predator into dying meat.

The essence of something that had been a worshipper at the altar of beauty and had killed itself for losing the ability to appreciate that which it valued above all else, tried to intercede after that. Its thoughts were deep and symphonic, and its counterattack gentle. It tried to deter the Hunter with compassion. But it, too, failed; and what was left of it when the Hunter was done was a corpse of shocking ugliness, incapable of singing anything but death.

In the end, Gordon couldn't have stopped them if he tried. They were all trapped, and they all had nothing to lose. They all fought for him, and they all lost; falling singly and together before the Hunter that would destroy anything to get to him.

In their mass sacrifice, Gordon Wilson learned something that once upon a time might have stopped him from placing that revolver in his mouth: that even at his loneliest, he had never been alone.

But by then there was nothing in the mix but the single greatest enemy either humanity or the ancestors of humanity had ever known, and Gordon Wilson, who had always been throughout his life one of the least of all men.

They faced each other: the Hunter in triumph, Gordon Wilson in dumbstruck silence. It didn't matter to either one of them that the battle was moot, that both combatants were just echoes of creatures that had already died; the only thing that mattered was a war that had been interrupted eons earlier, and that could only be finished by proxy, here and now.

And Gordon Wilson could hardly speak for laughing.

The worst kind of crash is the one that only seems to be taking place in slow motion—the one that wreaks so much damage all at once that time needs to telescope to accommodate it. The crash of the Travelers' bubble was like that. As it ping-ponged in and out of existence, at a trillion separate places throughout the universe, it skimmed the surface of a million separate worlds, flattening mountain ranges, boiling away atmospheres and annihilating civilizations. Carnage on such a scale had never happened before at any point in the history of creation. But each and every violent encounter also took its toll on the bubble itself—and by the time it ping-ponged across the Kcenhowten Confederacy, halving the population of that star-faring species in that instant, it was dented and powerless and leaking inverted singularities on all sides. It would have been doomed to destruction even if it still had fuel to slow its flight—and there was nothing; the little it still carried did not resemble despair at all.

It hurtled toward the end of everything, empty but for two ancient enemies who now faced each other for the very last time.

The Hunter snarled. *What are you laughing at?*

You, Gordon Wilson chortled, and had he been a living man instead of the intangible distilled essence of a suicide, he would have doubled over, clutching his ribs as he laughed so hard it hurt. It was the best kind of laughter—the kind that lights the places that have never known laughter before—and for the longest timc Gordon Wilson simply surrendered to it, thinking this the most glorious moment he had ever known. Near the end, he actually managed to speak: *You're such a fucking loser!*

I'm about to tear you to pieces.

Gordon whooped implacably. *Oh, yeah, I'm frightened. Give me a break. What the fuck are you going to do to me? Beat me up? Kill me? Stomp me to smithereens and piss on the smoking wreckage? In case you've missed the point, I'm already dead, you miserable pussy! I just put a bullet through my brain! I couldn't give less of a shit what* you *do to me! The most you can do is just put this little second-rate echo of me out of its misery, and you're not going to do that right away because that would leave you alone in here forever, with no way of getting out, and no way of ever going after anybody else! No, you're just going to stand right there and listen, while I say all the things that should have been said to you a long time ago!*

The Hunter trembled with rage. *Go ahead. Talk. It will amuse me to hear what you have to say.*

No it won't, Gordon said, as his laughter died and he faced the Hunter with the eyes of every person who'd ever lived. *It will shatter you. But I'll tell you anyway, because I don't like you very much. You know the people my people came from? The ones you hounded and harassed and pursued to the edge of extinction? I don't think they ever understood why you hated them so much. I don't think they ever understood why you needed to destroy them. I don't think it ever even occured to them to wonder. You were just a great unstoppable monster, annihilating them one world at a time, driving them back no matter how desperately they fought. And they never got around to asking why somebody as powerful as you would bother. But I know. It's because they scared you shitless.*

The Hunter roared his indignation in a voice loud enough to shatter continents. *Nonsense—*

And Gordon drowned him out with no difficulty at all, not with sheer volume, but with the simple confidence behind his words. *You were used to being the biggest baddest sonofabitch in the valley, weren't you? You were used to being the best, the strongest, the greatest. And then, all of a sudden, out of nowhere it seemed, along came this race of glorified monkeys, spreading from world to world with the speed of an explosion, and you wondered who they were and you took a close look and for the first time you saw something capable of challenging your ego. Because as primitive as they were, compared to you, and as weak as they were, compared to you, and as young as they were, compared to you, they had greater dreams, greater ambition, greater nobility, and greater potential, than a piece of shit like you could ever dream! And you just couldn't deal with it!*

The Hunter's voice took on the pathetic desperation of the loser who needs to assure himself he's won. *I still destroyed them all.*

Sure you did. Temporarily. But now we're back . . . still growing, still learning, still finding out what we can be. Our rise may be a little bumpier this time out, because of all the garbage you left us carrying around in our heads, but if anything that's only made us even stronger, and smarter, and faster, and better. I only wish I'd stuck around to see it.

The Hunter could have lashed out and sunk claws deep into Gordon's eyes and ribs and crotch and spine. He could have twitched his smallest finger and in an instant filleted Gordon from head to toe; he could have reduced Gordon to so many separate pieces of bloody shrapnel that there never would have been any way to tell what manner of creature he had been. None of it would have cost the Hunter any effort at all. But the Hunter did nothing.

Gordon Wilson smiled, faced down the embodiment of all of mankind's fears . . .

And, with a leer, gave him the finger.

The bubble was half-in, half-out of existence when it finally shattered. Its shrapnel popped into being on any number of worlds; they resembled nothing so much as shards of shattered mirror, capable of reflecting anything they saw. Some of the shards ended up on Earth, and some of the beings who found them were human: most notable among them an unhappy young woman named Tricia Winters, who found her fragment on the beach, stared into the oddly beautiful version of herself, and imagined for an instant that she saw a sadly contented little man smiling back. But that was the most anybody ever knew of the struggle that had been, for nobody anywhere in the known universe ever found a shard that reflected the Hunter.

As for the rest of it: the owner of the office-furniture shop found Gordon Wilson's automobile in his parking lot first thing Wednesday morning. After a properly respectful interval spent being violently and messily ill, he called the police, who called the medical examiner, who needed less than thirty seconds to pronounce the expected verdict of suicide. Everybody muttered the usual platitudes about the mess and the shock and the horrible waste of life; but nobody who looked at Gordon Wilson mentioned the triumph shining from eyes that should have been past showing any emotion at all.

JERUSALEM SYNDROME

Janet Berliner

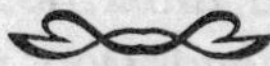

PETER STURNS' RETIREMENT PARTY WAS A GREAT SUCcess, partially because he was not in attendance. The people who had once loved the scientist, including Julie, his wife of some forty years, were only pretending to have a good time in case he returned in the middle of it all. In truth his absence was a great relief.

Especially to Julie.

She felt unburdened, slim, young, and optimistic—as if she had finally lost the excess weight that she had tried to lose for so many years. Every now and then she took out the note he had left and reread it, as if to reassure herself that her mind, at least, was still intact:

"Nothing personal, Julie, but I'm out of here," it read. *"Thanks for everything. Use my pension in good health. Marry Don or something."*

She looked outside the window at the red Porsche parked in the driveway. Peter had owned it for six years and she had not once been allowed to drive it. Now it was hers. He had left it behind and taken the ratty old station wagon, his checkbook, wallet, driver's license, a carton of cigarettes, and the contents of the liquor cabinet. Also a few clothes, his favorite books, a comforter, and a couple of pillows. And of course his camera equipment.

Not much to show for sixty-five years of life, Julie thought. Pathetically little, in fact.

"So where do you think he's gone, Julie?" their recently widowed friend, Don, asked.

Julie shrugged. "Who knows? Somewhere he can drink himself to death in peace, I guess." She turned away from the window, unwilling yet to voice the fact that at this moment she did not care.

Peter parked the old wagon at Monterey Airport, locked it carefully, and looked at his watch. There was an hour before the flight. Perfect timing, he thought. He could check in, have a drink, go outside for a smoke. When Julie was with him on trips, everything was done in a last-minute panic. This was to be his final lecture series, and he wanted to be on time. A week in Tel Aviv at the Technion, then back here, discard his suit, and drive to Cottonwood Cove.

He had discovered the cove quite by accident a year or so ago, after giving a lecture at UNLV. He loved Las Vegas for its very absurdity, loved it because there was no way to take yourself seriously in a city whose essence was built on dreams. But even as a man without religion, he sometimes found the city's godlessness disturbing.

So he had driven into the desert, seeking relief from the blanket of dreams that draped the city. And at the end of the stark and barren stretch of land that led from Searchlight down a winding road without street signs, he had found Cottonwood Cove.

The suddenness with which the water came upon him had left him breathless and as close to belief in a divinity as he had come in his adult years.

The inlet lay between Laughlin, Nevada, and Las Vegas, a small digression of the Colorado River. A trailer park, a funky motel. People who minded their own business. Paradise, in fact. He could happily die there.

Or live there.

He hadn't yet decided.

After a lifetime of obligatory decision-making, that felt best of all. There would be no more decision-making, no more thinking. He would live life by instinct; he would see the world through the lens of his camera and not even develop the photos if he didn't feel like it.

One flight took Peter to Los Angeles, the next one to New York. There he changed planes one more time and boarded the El Al flight to Tel Aviv. His sense of well-being did not evaporate until they were circling Lod Airport, and even then he knew that all he had to do was throw up and he'd be fine again. He had no one to blame except himself. El Al was a great airline; it was hardly the company's fault that he had eaten bagels and lox on top of far too many drinks during a too bumpy flight.

He stumbled out of the plane into the burning heat of the airport. On the ride in the sherut from Tel Aviv to Haifa his wish was granted and, much to the chagrin of the other passengers, he lost his breakfast. The driver took it all in stride.

He stopped in the middle of the desert, ordered Peter to take a walk, and tossed the contents of several water containers, which he apparently kept in the back of the vehicle for emergencies, over the offensive mess—saving enough to douse Peter before allowing him back into the minibus.

By the time Peter reached the students' quarters to which he had been assigned, he was feeling much better. He liked the simplicity of his room, which was spotlessly clean and contained nothing more than a narrow bed, a desk, and a bookcase that separated him from the space normally assigned to a second student. There was a bathroom for every two rooms, again, small but adequate. His meals were to be taken at the university itself, which was a fair walk through the relative coolness of a pine forest.

Peter was still drunk when he arrived at the Technion to give the first of his lectures on engineering techniques for the new millenium. Nobody seemed to care. They listened intently to everything he said, asked what seemed to him to be thousands of questions—most of them intelligent—and did not invite him to join them for any social events, for which lack he was sincerely grateful.

He made no excuses for his drinking. They only suggested, somewhat wryly it seemed to him, that he make certain to take in plenty of liquids. It was the only way to survive August in Israel, they said.

Someone did ask him if he was interested in seeing something of the country, to which question he responded with a resounding No.

This was his first time in Israel, but he'd long since stopped caring where he was when he gave his lectures, just so long as he had a comfortable bed, a bug-free room, and a plug for his computer so that he could stay in touch with his contacts through the Internet. Not that summers had ever been cool in Los Alamos, where he'd started his career, or in Searchlight, Nevada—a not-quite-town at the edge of the road near the turning to Cottonwood Cove—where he was going to retire.

The week in Israel passed quickly enough. Within a day, he'd shed his tie and rolled up the sleeves of his shirt. By the third day, he gratefully accepted a student's offer of a pair of shorts with which to replace his trousers. The little bit of sun that caught him between trees during his frequent walks back and forth to the main buildings was enough to give him a deep tan, but then he had always browned quickly. His white hair brightened into a halo, and only the drink-induced puffiness around his eyes betrayed his age and state of being.

Walking back to his room after his last lecture, Peter stopped to gather pine nuts. He placed them on a stone and cracked them open, savoring the wild smell and delicate flavor. He was tired of oranges and cheese and yogurt, with the occasional piece of chicken, cooked dry. He'd gone into the city a couple of times and eaten Arab food. For the most part an apolitical being, he was surprised to find that he felt a little guilty at enjoying it.

He was wondering whether he could get a few bags of nuts through the EPA inspection on the way home, when he blacked out.

Overnight case in one hand and videocam slung over his shoulder, Alex "Legs" Cleveland headed away from Don Laughlin's private airstrip toward the burgeoning town. Laughlin was, in more ways than one, the hottest town in the United States. By noon the temperature would be close to 130 degrees. He had several miles to walk, unless he thumbed a ride.

He could hear the CNN helicopter heading in for its landing. If he hurried, he could be in a comfortable room at Don Laughlin's Riverside Hotel in time to watch the first broadcast of the debacle he had created. A hot bath, a couple of stiff drinks, and he would feel a helluva lot more human.

He stepped around the dead bodies of the Zulu dancers he had brought from Bophututswana, ignored the security personnel who in turn ignored him, and thought briefly about his partner, Maury, sitting comfortably in his Beverly Hills office. He patted the video in his pocket. He had it all on tape: the Zulu war dance which had begun as a rehearsal and turned ugly; the slaughtering of black men and guards. Judging by the way O.J.'s video was selling, this one was good for at least a couple of million, more than enough to pay for the trip he had taken to Africa in search of something the same but different for the showrooms of Vegas.

Don Laughlin's private airstrip was in the Mojave Desert, on the outskirts of Laughlin, the southernmost town in Nevada, and right on the border of both California and Arizona. Hottest spot on earth where people actually lived. Rarely got below 125 in midsummer. Still it was close enough to Las Vegas to be somewhere in Alex's purview. He didn't want to go back to Africa. In fact, traveling anywhere was the last thing he wanted right now.

Well, maybe not the last. The last would be to go back to the Reservation.

If there were any place where Legs felt no sense of belonging, it was the Reservation.

What the hell. He had his credit cards and his lucky gemsbock horn in his pocket. He'd be all right.

He hopped a ride almost at once with a flatbed truck driver who was lonely for a bit of company.

"What you carrying?" Legs asked, settling down on the seat.

"Nothing yet. I'm on my way to Bullhead City to pick up a load of lumber for some crazy man down at the cove. He's building an ark, if you can believe that. Says he's Noah and the flood is coming." He shook his head. "Takes all sorts. Long as his money's A.D., I don't much care who he thinks he is."

Legs was half-drowsing after his night spent lying on a rock in the desert, so it took longer than usual for his entrepreneurial instincts to tune in to what the driver was saying.

"Say what?"

"Like I said. Man thinks he's Noah. Even dresses like someone out of a Heston movie. Went to Israel and caught this disease—"

"Disease?"

"My priest says it's called the Jerusalem Syndrome. Says it happens a lot, especially to people who aren't all that religious."

"So what's this disease? Is it contagious?"

"Don't guess so," the driver said. "Besides, he ain't hurting nobody. Just collecting animals, building an ark. Don't usually drive loads myself no more, but this I had to see."

"Like to see it myself," Legs said.

"Come with me if you like, I could use the company. Just want to get a quick breakfast and then I'm turning this load around. Fellow's been calling me every minute on my cell."

Legs fiddled with his camcorder, making sure there was room on the tape. Just in case. Hey, you never knew about these things. Maybe . . .

Maury would never believe this one if he told him, but if he had it on film . . .

Sitting in the shade of the small shelter he had built just feet from the shoreline, Peter waited for word from God with the same impatience with which he awaited the lumber. At his feet, open and held down at each corner by a rock, was the chart he had labored over by the light of a lantern.

The ark.

He opened a new bottle of the blackberry wine he had taken to drinking since his revelation and drank deeply, disregarding the red stream of liquid that added its design to the others on his robe and adhered to his beard. Propped against his side lay the walking stick he had whittled and over the corner of his canvas-backed director's chair hung the pair of binoculars he had traded for his camera at Super Pawn in downtown Vegas.

He picked them up, adjusted them, and stared out at the water. The alien Messiah was still out there, charging across the water of the inlet in a crazy, almost humorous sprint, with its legs windmilling around its ears at the rate of what Peter judged to be about twenty circles per second.

When the ark was built, the Messiah would speak to him, Peter thought. Maybe he too would learn to walk on water. In some vague part of his brain, he remembered a conversation he'd had with Tom McMahon at a Harvard tea in his student days. According to McMahon, the average creature would need to take 269 steps per second—per *second*—to walk on water.

A truck, moving too fast through the quiet area, roared to a stop behind him.

"Hey! You there! You Noah?"

Peter turned around. Waved. Smiled benignly and stood up. Two men descended from the truck, the driver and a balding middle-aged man with a videocam slung over his shoulder. Judging by his features, he was pure Navajo.

"Welcome," Peter said. "I am most pleased to see you." He looked at the driver and put out his hand. "You must be Zach. Thank you so much for bringing the lumber."

"Mind if I take your picture, um, Noah?" the Indian said. He stretched out a hand. "Alex 'Legs' Cleveland at your service. Just call me Legs."

"Later, Alex, when our work is done. I will even let you photograph Him." Peter pointed at the water.

"Now, allow me to help you with the lumber, gentlemen."

"Legs. Call me Legs," Alex said, his camera whirring.

Gently but firmly, Peter took the camera from Alex, turned it off, and placed it on his chair. "And you may call me Noah," he said.

"Crazy as a loon," Zach said, as soon as he and Legs were out of earshot.

"Or crazy as a fox." Legs opened his wallet and examined the contents, making sure that the driver saw the stack of hundred dollar bills inside. "Listen. Think you could take a couple of days off? I have an idea, but I'll need your help."

"Don't have another job scheduled for a few days," Zach said, glancing at the wallet. "Long as it's not illegal."

Legs laughed. "It's not illegal," he said. "But it is a little nuts."

"After *that,*" the driver nodded in Peter's direction, "anything'll seem normal. Where to, Gov'nor?"

"A telephone, a bar, a shower. Then a good night's sleep. Tomorrow we hustle. We're going to need a carny tent. T-shirts. Food." Legs pulled two bills out of his wallet.

Zach stared at them. "I got no idea what you're up to, but I got a feeling I oughta take a piece of the action. What *are* you up to?"

"Just the biggest thing since mother's milk." Legs leaned back and lit a cigarette. "Didn't you see what I saw?"

The driver shook his head.

"You didn't see Him, out on the water?"

Again Zach shook his head.

"Well, you're going to see it soon. Know anywhere we can copy the tape in my camcorder?"

"My place is the closest. Half an hour, at most."

"Fine. Put your foot flat. I'll pay for the ticket if you get one. We have be back before the CNN people leave the airstrip."

An hour or so later, they were back where Legs had started. He could see that Zach was squirrely about the whole thing. "Hey, listen," he said. "You can still walk away."

"It's just . . . well, what if it's really the Messiah. I been a church man all my life. Don't want to miss my chance for forgiveness by making money off of the Lord."

Damn Christian Fundamentalists, Legs thought. "Here." He labeled the dupe with his name and with Maury's, added the words, *Do not use for forty-eight hours,* and handed it to Zach. "Decide. In or out." He was ready to do a little praying himself. He could hardly walk out there and wait for someone to recognize him. His fortune was in Zach's hands.

Greed won out. "How d'you know they'll use it?"

"They'll use it. If *they* don't, *Hard Copy* will."

"What about money? Shouldn't they give us money?"

What's this "us" kemosabe, Legs thought. "Don't worry about money. This is free advertising. Move it, will you. Give me your cell code? I need to make a couple of calls while you're gone."

The first of which is to Maury, he thought. His partner would want to kill him—or have him certified. But the mention of money, big money, would tranquilize Maury.

It worked like a charm even—especially—in Beverly Hills.

For the next two days, Peter worked happily on laying out the wood for the foundation of the ark. Some of the locals, beginning to accept him, offered to lend a hand. None of them asked him why he was doing what he was doing, nor did he volunteer any information. The alien Messiah was nowhere to be seen, which did not concern Peter at all. He was yet to discover a pattern in His appearances.

Forty-eight hours after the delivery of the lumber, Legs and Zach returned, and Peter's idyllic lifestyle vanished. The minibuses arrived first, each one large enough to hold about ten adults. While a motley-looking group of people with cans of paint and brushes busied themselves with painting, "$1 per ride to see the Alien Messiah" on the sides of the busses. Legs supervised the setting up of T-shirt and food stands and a row of portajohns. News helicopters hovered overhead: ABC, NBC, CBS. Inevitably, CNN arrived on the scene. Reporters with cameras and newspads badgered him for interviews, and a publisher—flanked by two people who introduced themselves respectively as agent and lawyer—offered him an obscenely large amount of money for exclusive rights to his story.

He took no notice of any of them until one of them,

a kid the age of Peter's grandson, offered him a full bottle of bourbon. He turned out to be from *Rolling Stone*. Peter took the bottle, thanked the young man, and politely offered him a drink, which he took.

"So where's your Messiah?" the kid asked.

"Out there somewhere," Peter said.

"How big is he? Looked pretty small to me."

"Who guaranteed big?" Peter asked. "Everything looks small out on the water. Just think about the real size of a porpoise and how small it looks from the deck of a ship. Tell me, kid, when did you see Him?"

"On CNN."

Peter glanced across at Legs. He couldn't really blame the man for cashing in on this, and he didn't have the energy to get angry, but he wished like hell that this hadn't happened. The only people—outside of Legs and Zach and the newspeople—who showed no resentment were the owners of the little motel. And why shouldn't they be happy, Peter thought. Probably the first and last time that their motel would get this kind of attention. Until they made the movie, he thought wryly. Produced and directed, no doubt, by Alex "Legs" Cleveland.

"What animals will you put in the ark first, Mr. Noah," the kid asked, slurring his words.

"Whatever comes along," Peter said. Snakes, he thought. Deadly snakes. May they off the lot of you. "Legs! Zach!" He left his chair and stumbled toward them. "Any way to stop this, you bastards?"

Legs shook his head. "I'm sorry," he said.

"Sure you are!" Suddenly he started to laugh. He

held out the bottle. "Oh well. We all have to make a living somehow."

"Want me to drive for a while?" Don said.

"No, thanks." Julie glanced at him and smiled as she saw his white-knuckled grip on the window-frame.

The red Porsche appeared to defy gravity as it speeded its way toward Cottonwood Cove. Small wonder Peter hardly ever gave me any, she thought, resting her hand lightly on the gear shift. He got all the excitement he needed out of this thing. Feels like driving on whipped butter.

"We'll need to get him help right away," she said. "I set up an appointment with Ed for tomorrow morning."

"Ed's as crazy as Peter," Don said.

"Maybe." Or maybe neither of them was crazy, she thought. Maybe she and Don were the crazy ones, living their lives by the rules as if it mattered.

Up ahead, right about where a sign said Cal-Nev-Ari—a town consisting of a trailer park on one side of the highway and a barn and a general store on the other—they had to slow down. The traffic was not quite bumper-to-bumper, but it was heavy enough.

"Where the hell are all of these people going?" Julie asked.

Don reached over and switched on the radio. They listened together in silence to the special report about the goings on in Cottonwood Cove.

"Traffic is completely backed-up all the way from Searchlight," the newscaster said. "Watch for over-heating, folks."

"Maybe he really has found God," Julie said.

"For Chrissakes, Julie. That was a Jesus lizard on the water. Not some alien Messiah like they're saying."

"Uh-huh." She glanced at herself in the rearview mirror and reached up to tidy her hair. She couldn't quite figure out her own emotions. It had been three months since she had seen Peter, spoken to him. Yet it wasn't until she'd seen him on the screen that she'd realized that she missed the son-of-a-bitch. With any luck at all, seeing him in person would cure that.

A sign at the side of the road said fifteen miles to go. At this rate, it would take all day to get there. In the distance, she could see colored balloons floating in the sky and a blimp with a banner that read, "Come and greet the alien Messiah." She and Don had started from Monterey within an hour of the CNN broadcast. The drive should have taken nine or ten hours. It was sixteen hours before they left the car in a large roped-off section of the desert, bought hot dogs and lemonade from a kid at the side of the road, and flagged a dollar-a-piece ride to the cove.

"What do we do if he won't come with us?" she asked, hanging on to Don's arm.

"Leave without him, I suppose. He's over twenty-one."

"All these people," she said. "They look so serious. They really believe, don't they?"

Don shrugged. "Most of the people in the world are stupid."

Just shows how desperately they need to believe in something, Julie thought, but she didn't say it for fear he would laugh at her. She had always hated being laughed at. But not Peter. Peter didn't care about things like that.

Perhaps that was why he had left her.

Or why he believed.

That he did believe was clear from the tape. Why else would he have called himself Noah, and be building an ark, and speak with such reverence of the creature he called the alien Messiah?

The bus was overcrowded and smelled of sweat and anticipation. Someone had begun to sing "Onward Christian Soldiers" and, softly, the others joined in.

Julie found herself humming with them.

Quickly, she switched to "Hatikvah." No one around her seemed to mind. As the final chorus of their song ended, they took up hers.

She was singing the last verse when the bus stopped and she spotted Peter. He was sitting on a director's chair in the dirty robes he had worn on the tape, staring out at the water. Young people sat at his feet. To his left stood a broad-shouldered, serious-looking man who looked like a truck-driver; on the other side stood an aging Navajo who wore a broad grin. Near the water, a crowd of people of all ages built the foundations of a large wooden structure.

"The ark," Julie said. "They're really building an ark."

She stepped down from the bus and looked out across the water. The Jesus lizard they had seen on television was nowhere to be seen. The whole thing reminded her of Woodstock, she thought. Not the bad part of Woodstock, but the good part. The joining together, the camaraderie, the belief that rose tangibly into the air and spoke of hope for the future.

She looked around at the faces of the people gathered here, and turned to look at the crowds who pressed to join them. Tugging at Don's arm, she pulled him back toward the road and the Porsche and home.

She stopped in her tracks. Taking the keys of the Porsche out of her pocket, she handed them to Don. "Here, you take them," she said. "Drive the car home. It's yours." She turned around to face the water. "You're crazy, Peter," she yelled happily.

Stripping off her stockings, she twirled around on her bare feet. As she broke into the chorus of a song whose title she no longer remembered, one from her distant youth, she realized that it didn't matter whether the thing out on the water, Peter's alien Messiah, was an overgrown basilisk lizard that used air bubbles to support its weight on the water, or some creature from outer space, or even if it was God.

It really didn't matter at all.

THE END OF THE DREAM TIME

Catherine Mintz

THAT'S WHAT I BROUGHT YOU TO SEE. THAT BIG GRAY honeycomb the air makes a little noise in as it passes through. It's an eerie old thing to look at, isn't it? But maybe it looks like just another wind-carved rock to you, not that different from half the stuff up at this end of the canyon.

Bet you wonder why I had you walk all this way in the heat when we could have talked sitting in the shadow of the council house or out in the low fields digging roots with the rest. But I've brought all the children of the families here to see it, and now it's your turn.

Well, sit down in the shade while I have my say, and then we'll go back.

Look at it. I've been up here on windy days when it howled like it was alive and in pain. Winter nights, sometimes, when there's a storm from the west you can hear it in the village, so far away you'd take it for a feral dog if you didn't know.

Any of your cousins ever talk to you about it? No? Well, we kind of keep the knowing for the grown-ups. One day it'll be worn away. I don't know what they'll point to for warning then. Maybe it won't matter.

It was different here once. There was more water in the creek, and plants grew wild all along the canyon. Every spring all the young ones had to go out and pull them by the handfuls to make sure the corn reached its full height.

We hated it—it left you tired at night, and your hands got all green with the sap. It was a good life, even though I was too young to know it. Things were good here, better than the best season you've ever seen, or are likely to see.

Maybe so. I wouldn't mind being wrong.

Let me get on with this. It was my cousin Georgiana who saw it first. She was more spirited than most, a good worker, although some grown-ups called her flighty. When she'd pulled enough weeds . . .

They're the plants you don't want.

Nothing, just throw them away to dry up.

I said, things were different.

As I was saying, when she'd pulled enough weeds to satisfy Old Farnam—he was in charge of this section of farms . . .

We had fields right up through here and beyond, clear up to the Whitson's gap.

Yep. Well, when Georgiana'd pulled enough to feel sure she could satisfy Farnam that she was entitled to a break, she climbed up on the rim, right there, where there's a notch.

No particular reason, I expect. Just to look around. There'd be a bit more of a breeze up there, and you could see the hawks hunting, riding the wind up from the canyon, watching the rim grass for rabbits and snakes.

Something like a quail, but they ate . . .

Now I want you to listen to this and not keep interrupting me. I'll explain things like that after. There's enough hard ideas coming without picking away at the meaning of this word and that.

Georgiana was up there, looking around, maybe flipping a pebble or two back into the river, when she saw a cloud, flying across the wind, coming from the Black Mountains.

That way.

Well, we'd have to climb up there.

Not today.

Maybe when it's cooler.

If you can get him to, it's all right with me, but we're not doing it right now.

Don't you go sulky on me. This is important. You're always wanting to be more grown-up, now's your chance.

No, she couldn't tell what it was. Georgie just knew it wasn't anything that should be where it was, doing what it was, and it was coming right at her, fast. I suppose if she'd had time she would have skinned down out of there and run home, but she didn't.

She hunkered down in the rocks right there in that notch.

I said, if Tim'll take you, you can go, but not with

me, and not today. I'm too stiff in the joints to go climbing around for no reason.

Well, *I've* seen it, and I'm telling you about it.

That thing came gusting in and settled right there where the honeycomb is, but it didn't look like that then. It looked like—see that cloud over there, the one with two bumps on top and a flat bottom?—like that, but solid, like cotton fluff. A clever thing. We probably wouldn't have noticed it if Georgiana hadn't happened to have been there.

I've always wondered if it mightn't have been around for a while.

Well.

Georgie said the whole thing just sat there, shimmering, for a little while, then sort of oozed in on itself and turned into big sky-boulder, as pitted and black as the piece in the council house. She could not believe her eyes, and she wasn't about to go up to the thing and touch it. Might be something dangerous. She got herself back down, quiet as a mouse, and ran for home.

We all came up and had a look at it.

We didn't trust it. It was unnatural. Who'd believe an enormous rock like that would fall out of the sky without making a sound, or leaving a hole in the ground bigger than our village? Grandfather's cousin, Jay Hmoung, said a meteor that size should have left bits and pieces behind it for a day's walk and more. We searched all around and found nothing . . .

I think maybe something was already inside, watching. Gives me a funny feeling to think about it now. I was one of the boys set to hunt around it, up close, looking for scorch marks, or burns, or anything that would show that huge thing hadn't just been set in place, like an egg on a tabletop.

I wasn't scared. I should have been—would have been, if I had any sense—but I wasn't.

I believe you. But sometimes it's better to be a little frightened.

Okay. There it was, and there it sat, and we were sure it wasn't natural, but we couldn't figure how, what, and why it had come to be. It worried everybody for a while, even if they didn't believe Georgiana's story.

Oh, yeah, there were plenty of doubters.

A lot figured she'd been asleep, hadn't noticed the stone when she climbed into the notch, then, confused by the changes when she woke up, half-dreamed what she told us. A few said she'd lied to cover up that she'd been sleeping, even though she wasn't on watch. Almost nobody wanted to believe she'd told the simple truth.

They didn't mean any harm. It was just a more comfortable sort of thought. You get older and find out people mostly don't like to face strange things. A cloud that turned into a rock . . .

Well, maybe you won't. I hope not. Someone has to do some thinking around here.

Even if we weren't all that happy about it, there was always work to do. We went back to the business of scratching a living, and everything went along about the way it always had. For a while.

I was getting old enough that they expected me to help with the hunting. I didn't mind. I was good at it, and it was like a day off. If I made it back with six rabbits or so, or a dozen quail, they counted it time well spent, no matter what I'd done with the rest of the day.

Nope, that wasn't even very many. There was more water then. A hunter could count on finding small game. It was a bad night when we didn't have meat in camp.

Yeah, well, so do I. So do I. Some nights we had a half a rabbit apiece—could have had more, but it would have been a waste. We ate green corn, then, too. Didn't wait for the harvest.

Just planted a bit more, is all.

I know.

I told you, I was out hunting. It was no accident that I doubled over to here. Farnam liked us to keep a eye on the thing, and we mostly made a point of just happening by, if it wasn't too far out of our way.

So I was the first to see it.

You should have wanted to know that already. Ask important questions first. Suppose it *was* dangerous, there might be something you needed to do.

Remember when you learned to sling stones? You had to learn how to pick out a pebble and how to hit something. Then you had to learn how to find a rabbit? Then you had to learn how to hit a rabbit. Learning how to handle an emergency is something like that. You have to learn all the pieces . . .

All right, I'll get on with it.

When I came near the rock I could see that there was something moving around outside, picking up bits of this and that and putting them down again. I dropped flat on my belly in the bushes.

It hadn't. I don't know why. I hadn't been especially careful, just come jogging in with my back load of rabbits, wanting to take a quick look and get on back to the village. It *should* have seen me . . .

It was as big as that boulder over there, the brown one I could just about touch the top of if I stood real tall.

It wasn't ugly. If it had looked more like us, I might have thought it was, but rabbits, quail, and snakes are just themselves. This was like that. Just something else. Six-legged. Or four-legged if you counted the things it stood on as legs, and called the other pair arms. There's drawings in the council house. You'll see them.

I crawled all the way to the second rim gap on my stomach, then got up and ran to tell Old Farnam. He told the headwoman . . .

It was a woman in those days.

Your mother has a lot to teach you if you think that.

Time will tell. Her name was Shirilee, and she got all the elders together fast as she could. It didn't take long before they decided the first thing they needed was more information. They sent me back.

I wasn't scared the first time, but the second time I'd listened to what the council members said to one another. They sure weren't making any assumption that whatever-it-was was friendly. It was an open secret that the elders knew a good bit they didn't talk about, kept things from the youngers.

So we wouldn't grow up afraid, I suppose.

I'm telling you now.

There wasn't anything stirring outside when I crept up, but what looked like a meteor had changed into the honeycomb you can see up there. Look at it. See all the hollow places, bigger than a tall man?

They were capped and closed, each filled with things like the first whatever-it-was I'd seen, except they were all small, soft-looking, and white.

I took my time watching. Presently I was sure there was nothing stirring, and I got up and went walking around, not at all worried about the thing I'd seen. I was feeling pretty bold, looking forward to having the elders' attention when I told my story.

Until I nearly stepped on it. Or what was left of it. Skin, mostly. It was lying there on the ground like an old worn-out glove, sagging in on itself. The bottle-flies were at it already, and the crows had eaten the eyes.

It hummed and heaved and shifted a bit. For a moment, I thought it was a alive like that. Made my stomach turn over. I nearly retched my guts up, crouching in the shade of the nearest bush, too sick to find better cover. When I finished, I looked up . . .

No, I'm all right.

When I looked up, all those soft white things had turned in their cells, and they were all staring at me. All those pale, blind-looking eyes, watching, watching *me*.

I ran so fast I didn't even know I'd cut my foot right through my moccasin until I got back to the village. When I finished babbling everything to the elders, they didn't even bother to vote, just started out for here without another word, even though it was near dark.

I couldn't go with them, but everyone who could came up here that very night, and gathered every bit of dry wood and brush they could find. Made a pile taller than a tall man, all the way around.

Set fire to it.

The cells popped in the heat, and the things inside came out writhing, fell down into the fire, tried to crawl out, died sizzling. Everything but that stony bit up there could burn, and did, burned for three nights and two days. We kept guards on it all that time, and the young ones ran back and forth, bringing firewood.

I was a little bit of a hero.

Until the next rains didn't come.

See, one of the things the eldest hadn't even told the elders was exactly how we came to be here. You've sung the song yourself, so you know that, time was, we were up there among the stars, traveling to new homes.

I don't know, I was never there myself. I'm telling you what they told me. It was a big fight, us and them, out there between here and some other place. We never saw who they were. Maybe we lost and maybe we won, but the boat we were on . . .

Like Jay's skiff, but bigger, and closed.

Metal, I think.

The *Illyrion.*

That's a *name,* not a thing.

We—not us of course, but our great-great's and great-great-great's—crashed down yonder. They expected to be killed by the fall, but they skidded in, every one knocked out cold. When they found they were alive they came out of their boat . . .

Oh, it was big, bigger than three or four council houses all made into one.

They came out of their boat to have a look around. It was pretty badly smashed, so they carried a good deal of what they had out, planning to shelter in a cave, use some of the boat's metal for a big panel to close it off.

That's right, the big one in the east cliff. They never did make that door. When they were all out, the *Illyrion* exploded for no reason they could figure out. Vaporized is more like it. There was almost nothing left. They were stuck . . .

Jay'll tell you more about that, some other time. That's his part of the story. I'm telling you my part.

Every one of us can recite some of it, so we won't forget.

Now I want you to listen to me carefully. At first, they thought they had just been lucky to survive, and luckier still they'd moved enough stuff out of the *Illyrion* that they could do a little farming and even have enough to eat while they waited for the crops to bear.

They had hopes that one of the other star-boats would come and take them away, back to where they came from, or on to where they were going. But time went by, and what with one thing and another, they gave up on that. Mostly the oldest just died out and their hopes died with them.

If the eldest thought they were just fortunate, their youngers weren't so sure, especially once they saw *that* thing. It got talked about. It might have been one of *them,* the ones that shot us down. Might have.

We talked about it a lot. Some of us began to wonder if maybe we were put here. To be watched. By the whatever-it-was. Maybe when it died, none of the rest of them wanted to bother . . .

It's a hard idea, I know.

You're shivering, you've heard enough for one day. Let's go back now. Mind you, you're not to scare your youngers with this. They'll never grow up venturesome if they hear it too early. That's why we wait. We have to stay strong.

No, that's the whole story. The rest's just details. You'll come to know them like the rest of us. Any ideas you have, well, tell us. We've tried most things, but a fresh mind is always welcome.

Maybe it's just a silly notion, and everything's been a happenstance. Maybe the rains will come next season, and you'll see a hawk hunting quail in the rim grass, and we'll all eat green corn and rabbit until our bellies ache, and wonder why we worried so.

Just don't bet on it.

REALIZATIONS

Don D'Ammassa

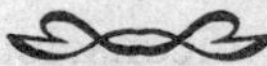

WHEN HER FATHER ADMITTED HE WAS COLOR BLIND, Connie immediately wanted to see what the world looked like through his eyes.

"You mean reds and greens are all backward?" She was ten years old.

"Not exactly. They're just not the same and sometimes I can't tell one shade from another."

"Then what colors *do* you see?"

She hadn't understood that their frames of reference could be so different that the question was meaningless.

Almost twenty years later, she faced the same problem on an even greater scale.

"Are you all right, Dr. Jensen?"

Connie raised her head and pushed back from the console. "Yes, just tired."

"Can I get you some coffee?"

"That would be fine, Margery." She wouldn't drink it, just wanted to dismiss the technician without offending her.

The last message from Rikashi was still on the screen, just as impenetrable as ever.

"You are unusually purple today, Connie Jensen. You should kill someone softly."

"Lovely sentiment." A male voice spoke from the back of the room.

Connie blinked, disoriented, glanced over her shoulder. Colin Kraft had entered the interview room with his usual unconscious stealth.

"You're anthropomorphizing again, Colin." Kraft was ostensibly a White House liaison, but everyone knew he worked for the NSC. Rikashi had only mentioned him once in his messages, an offhand reference to "the oblique one with the scoured mind." It made more sense than most of the alien's communications, which probably meant they understood even less than they thought they did.

"Colin is here if you wish to speak to him," she typed.

A new row of characters etched themselves onto the screen. "Duality endures. Opportunity for fulfillment offers itself. Do you grasp?"

Kraft eased into the adjacent chair without an invitation. He had from time to time made casual sexual advances to Connie, but she had sensed his underlying disinterest. In a moment of insight, she'd realized he was sexless, adopting the pose as part of his mask.

"Still looks pretty random to me. Maybe our first

alien visitor is insane. Maybe that's why so much of what it says is meaningless." He glanced at the upper monitor, a segmented screen showing the alien's living quarters from four separate views. Rikashi stood at the computer terminal, his vaguely human-shaped body covered with millions of tiny cilia that moved as though they had individual life. Every few days he shed about 5 percent of them. New growth reached maturity within a week.

"Not at all. He just recognized your arrival and suggested that I murder you to reduce my purpleness. And we've established that Rikashi is male, Colin, not an 'it.'" More or less, anyway. The exchange was just play-acting. Connie had no doubt at all that Kraft had personal access to every progress report she and the rest of the staff turned in, and probably their private notes as well.

"Charming fellow. Wish we knew how it sensed our comings and goings. Do you suppose it's telepathic?"

"There's no evidence supporting that hypothesis."

Dr. Schroeder had asked that very question, and Rikashi had replied, "Darkness illuminates." Maybe he could see through the walls.

"Anything new from the recovery team?"

"How would I know? According to CNN they haven't found anything but insignificant fragments scattered across the ocean floor."

"Your mind is pink but your lips are blue." It slipped out before she realized it.

Kraft frowned. "Is that supposed to mean something."

"No, just thinking aloud." She turned back to the

screen, satisfied that she'd called the man a liar as Rikashi might have done, and even more satisfied to know he'd read her interpretation of that phrase in her last report.

He said nothing when he left a moment later and Connie didn't watch him go.

"Release flees sideways to your future. I taste salt and sour and the air moves fitfully."

Connie checked the telltales quickly, fearing something had gone amiss with the environmental controls, but they hadn't varied. Rikashi could survive Earth's atmosphere but he was more comfortable with a lower proportion of oxygen and a different mix of trace elements. Could he be referring to her own breathing?

"Understanding remains elusive. We value life and will not take another for small reason."

"You must realize life's changes never end. To restore balance is a grand endeavor. We are red together in our sweet bones and flesh, Connie Jensen. Your time is always within my mind."

Connie chose to interpret that as a compliment. She needed one desperately.

"This situation is unacceptable!" Paul Mitchelson was theoretically the head of the contact team, although everyone knew that Kraft—currently sitting quietly in a corner—was pulling or, more frequently, jerking the strings. "The creature is obviously intelligent, speaks English fluently, never sleeps, and is always willing to communicate. You've had four months to study it, and the only facts we're certain of could be summarized on a single page."

Connie felt no impulse to defend herself, but Julian Ngambo was clearly upset and spoke without being recognized.

"You underestimate the difficulties, Mr. Director. This isn't some isolated human tribe we're dealing with here. Rikashi comes from a totally different culture, a different biology and psychology. We're not even sure that language serves the same function with his people that it does with humans. There have been indications that these beings may possess some temporal sensory abilities—"

Mitchelson cut him off impatiently. "If the creature could travel in time, why doesn't it hop back to its ship and prevent it from crashing in the first place?"

Connie sighed. No one had implied Rikashi could travel in time physically, but there was some evidence that the alien occasionally responded to events that had not yet taken place, or which had happened weeks earlier. Unofficially they were calling it the Vonnegut Effect.

The meeting ended with increasingly strident exhortations to achieve a breakthrough. "In case it escaped your attention, at least four more escape pods entered the Earth's atmosphere, and three of them came down in China. I don't have to tell you what could happen if the Communists steal a march on us, do I?"

Someone was slumped in the corridor, leaning against the door to her apartment. Connie hesitated. The nights were growing colder in Virginia and while Maclean didn't have a large homeless population, they were around if you looked for them. She couldn't resent anyone wanting to come inside where it was warm, but she also needed to get into her apartment, and her bed, before she dropped from exhaustion.

"Excuse me, please?" She tried to sound both friendly and firm as she extended the key toward the door. The figure beneath her stirred, raised its head.

"Sarah? What are you doing here?"

"Came to visit," her eighteen-year-old sister answered sullenly. "I had to get out of that place."

Connie bit back the first words that came to mind, unlocked the door, and led the way inside.

"Does Uncle Bob know where you are?"

Sarah rolled her eyes. "I'm fine, sis, thanks for asking. No, he doesn't know. If I'd left him a note, he'd've been here waiting for me."

"I'm going to call him right now." She started to fish around in her purse for her address book, but Sarah snatched it away.

"Wait . . . one . . . minute!" The younger girl was clearly furious. "At least give me a chance to tell you my side of the story first."

I really don't need this, Connie told herself, not right now. "All right, let's sit and talk."

"I can't live there anymore, Connie. I just can't. I'm not going back. They don't want me there anyway."

"Don't talk nonsense. Uncle Bill volunteered to take us in when Mom and Dad died, you know. No one made him do it."

"I realize that." Sarah bit her lip, averted her eyes. "But ever since . . . you know . . . it hasn't been the same. I don't think he ever forgave me for running off and . . . and everything. And since he and Mary got married last year, well, it's just like I don't belong there any more."

"But that's your home now, Sarah. Where else can you go?"

Sarah faced her again, eyes brittle with tears. "I thought maybe I could stay with you for awhile. Sleep on your couch, clean house for you." She gestured vaguely at the chaos of the apartment, dirty dishes on the counters, newspapers tossed into corners, dirty laundry populating small colonies around the furniture. "Not that you need it or anything." A ghost of a smile, quickly gone. "And I could look around for a job. I'm eighteen, Connie. It's time for me to start living again."

"What about Doctor Martin? She's been very good for you."

"Yeah, I guess so. But she says I have to start doing the healing myself, that I'm using her to avoid dealing with my future. I think she's right."

They talked some more and eventually Connie called their uncle and told him Sarah would be staying with her for a few weeks. She thought he was more relieved to hear that than he had been to discover his niece was safe.

Rikashi never slept so the interview rooms were staffed around the clock. Connie swapped with Dr. Kelso for the graveyard shift for a few days because she suspected that the alien's behavior fluctuated diurnally even though the habitat was isolated from the outside world.

That's how she happened to be on duty when the alarms went off.

They had just completed another puzzling exchange in which she'd tried to learn the reason his people had come to Earth's system. Rikashi kept repeating that "the purpose of life is change" and "the purpose of change is life," and insisted that Connie's purple was growing deeper. She was reviewing the transcript when lights began flashing and a buzzer sounded.

Instinctively she glanced at the monitor, saw Rikashi unfold his two-meter-tall body from where it crouched in one corner.

A mature tabby cat stepped out from between the alien's legs and began to clean itself.

Dr. Irving burst into the room, pointing at the screen. "Do you see that, Connie? Where the hell did that come from? The security people are going to shit bricks!"

Connie watched, fascinated, as Rikashi approached the cat. The animal showed no sign of alarm, not even when those writhing, cilia-covered arms wrapped around its body.

"Do you suppose he's going to eat it?"

"Why would he? We supply all the food he wants, and with the right chemical structure."

"Maybe he wants dessert."

The cat was almost invisible now, completely enfolded by the cilia but showing no sign of panic. Rikashi bent his body forward slowly, obscuring the animal completely, then straightened up.

The cat was gone, as if it had never been there in the first place.

"First of all," Mitchelson said quietly, "it was not an hallucination. Hallucinations don't show up on film." The oversized screen flashed, then replayed the cat's brief visit to the isolation chamber. "Security has gone over the facility in great detail and we are satisfied that the integrity of the containment area was not breached by any conventional means." He paused a moment to let that sink in.

"If there was any doubt at all in your minds about the urgency of solving this problem before our friends in China do, or even our supposed German friends for that matter, I trust this will erase it."

Margery inclined her head toward Connie and whispered clandestinely. "I guess we can take that as confirmation of the rumor that the Germans recovered the missing pod."

But Connie wasn't paying attention. She was thinking about the brief exchange she'd had before security pulled everyone out of the complex for debriefing.

"Where did the cat come from, Rikashi?" She'd typed the words with trembling fingers, backspacing twice to correct mistakes.

"Life's potential is in all places. Life's purpose is life's purpose."

The session lasted through the morning and into the afternoon. By the time they called it quits for the day, Connie was afraid she'd nod off on the drive home.

Sarah kept the apartment neat and orderly, laundered, cleaned, cooked, did the shopping, and ran errands. She had even found a part-time job running a cash register at a nearby convenience store. After her initial uneasiness, Connie discovered she was glad her sister had come, even though it saddened her to see how much of the old fervor for life had not returned.

Sarah had run away from home with her boyfriend while sixteen. Jimmy Nicholson was a charmer, good looking, well spoken, obviously intelligent, but underneath he was petty, cruel, and thoughtless. They were living in Boston when she got pregnant, apparently to her great delight. She wrote to Connie several times, her letters filled with enthusiastic plans for the baby, but never provided a return address.

When she was eight months pregnant, she and Nicholson had a violent argument. He broke her jaw, her nose, and her right arm, and while she was lying unconscious on the floor, he had kicked her repeatedly in the abdomen, then took off, never to be heard from again. Sarah had almost bled to death. She lost the baby and was told that there was no possibility of her ever having another.

Connie still felt her eyes begin to sting whenever she thought about it.

"How'd your day go? Catch any spies?"

"Half a dozen before lunch. Only three in the afternoon. What's for supper?" Connie felt awkward not being able to tell her sister, or anyone else for that matter, about her current assignment, but Sarah didn't seem to resent being kept in the dark.

"Just spaghetti. Sorry, but I didn't have time to do

anything more complicated. I was out with Mrs. Wentworth all day."

"Mrs. Wentworth from downstairs? What's her problem?"

"Cat got out somehow. She was worried sick and she's so frail, I didn't want to let her roam the neighborhood alone. This isn't the best part of town, if you hadn't noticed."

"Did you find it?"

"The cat? Yeah, it was back in her apartment when we gave up. I guess it found a great new place to hide because I looked all over with her before we went out."

Connie felt a sudden, intense pain in the center of her forehead. "What kind of cat is it?"

"Oh, just a tabby."

Rikashi spent three hours the following morning misunderstanding, or deflecting, her questions about the cat. "Life is a continuum, Connie Jensen. Potentiality transcends physical limitations. You must realize this."

"So the cat can be anywhere at all, at any time at all?"

"Only if you realize its existence."

She shook her head with frustration, stretched her arms above her head, glanced back through the last few exchanges, still visible on the screen. Something almost made sense. Rikashi had emphasized several times that she needed to realize the nature of the situation, and she had responded that she was trying to. But suddenly another interpretation suggested itself.

With a few keystrokes, she did a simple search and replace, then sent the transcript to the print queue. As the pages dropped into the bin, she read each in turn, searching for the word *realize,* which was now underlined and italicized wherever it appeared.

"Oh my God," she whispered.

"If this is your idea of a joke, Dr. Jensen, I am not amused." Mitchelson slammed his desk drawer shut and turned away, obviously dismissing her. But Colin Kraft spoke up from the corner.

"I'd like to hear her out, Dr. Mitchelson."

"It's not as farfetched as it may sound. Look, no two of us live in the exact same world, and we're human. How can we expect a nonhuman life-form to do so?"

"We interpret the real world differently, but that doesn't mean there isn't a single objective truth." Mitchelson was still surly, but in deference to Kraft he'd modulated his tone.

"In one sense, perhaps. But a color-blind person's vision is just as valid as our own, it just isn't the majority. For some people, chocolate tastes great, or spicy cooking, or broccoli. Some people see the world as a wonderful, beautiful place to live, others as a Darwinian rat race, still others as a dangerous environment filled with sinister plots and evil forces." She forced herself not to look at Kraft as she said this last. "Each of those interpretations might be equally valid. Rikashi's species realizes how the universe works."

"So you're saying that these aliens know the truth and we don't?"

She shook her head. "You're making the same mistake I did. When Rikashi told me I had to realize the truth, I thought he was criticizing my understanding. But he uses the word *realize* in the sense of 'making real.' If the laws of the universe aren't absolute, if they're malleable, then perhaps we can pick and choose which of those laws to . . . to realize."

Mitchelson dismissed her moments later, clearly convinced she'd gone off the deep end. But Kraft remained silent, thoughtful, and Connie wondered if he had more imagination than she'd given him credit for.

"Conversance with the brother of your womb home would be desirable."

Connie stared at the screen thoughtfully. "I have no brother. Do you mean my sister?"

"The one whose greater purple stains your own. Slow tears in the peaceful darkness."

"How do you know about Sarah? I've never mentioned her to you."

"The potential for that knowledge has always existed. It has only now reached realization."

Tumblers clicked in her mind. "I have always had the ability . . ." she backspaced over the last word and replaced it, "potential to tell you, therefore you possess the knowledge. Is that it?"

"If that is your realization."

She pondered that. "Then why haven't you ever asked me what has happened to your surviving shipmates?"

"Where there is no potential, there is no realization." There was a pause. "Because you will never know what has happened to them."

"And do you?"

"I realize that they will continue. The shape of that continuity has many branches."

"Could you have saved your ship? Could you have prevented it from crashing?"

"Yes." There was a long pause. "But we didn't realize it in time."

Three days later, Rikashi escaped.

Kraft and the security chief, a wafer-thin man named Lofton, met Connie in one of the small meeting rooms.

"What's up? I have lots of work to do today."

"I think you'll find your schedule has been altered, Miss Jensen." Lofton stared at a sheaf of papers, never met her eyes.

"That's Dr. Jensen," she said quietly. "Altered how?"

"Have you observed any change in the subject's behavior during the past few days . . . Dr. Jensen?"

"Nothing in particular. Why?"

Lofton looked stubborn but Kraft seemed to shake himself awake. "We've got a problem, Connie. It escaped about an hour ago."

"It? You mean Rikashi? Escaped? How could he escape from a sealed room?"

Lofton looked uncomfortable, Kraft mildly amused. "A wire burned out in the primary alarm system, and someone spilled coffee onto the backup and shorted it. A few seconds later the magnetic lock on the door malfunctioned for as yet undetermined reasons. The guard at station one was tying his shoelace and looked away from the door for less than ten seconds. The main security monitor burned out and the secondary wasn't live for almost fifteen seconds. The corridor guard was using the restroom and his relief was reading a magazine. Several other minor coincidences contributed as well."

"So he's out of the compound?"

"Yes, it seems so. We thought you might possibly know how he managed all this. The chain of circumstance is, you must admit, extremely unlikely."

"Unlikely," she said slowly, "but possible. And I guess today Rikashi realized how to escape."

The apartment was empty when she got home. Connie picked at some leftovers, too uneasy to eat. Where could Rikashi have gone, and for what reason? She replayed their last several interviews in her mind, searching for some clue, ended up with a headache and no insights.

It was almost ten o'clock. Where was Sarah?

Connie opened the door to the guest room, wondering if her sister had left a note. The room was neat and orderly, no messages in sight, nothing out of place except for something spilled on the rug beside her bed. She crouched, examined the spill. Inch-long fibers, tubular, dark.

Rikashi's molted cilia.

Something's happened to Sarah, she realized, then mentally backtracked in a panic. The last thing she should do is realize any such thing. Realizations were dangerous now.

She called Colin Kraft at his emergency number.

Sarah was missing for four days. More of the cilia had been found in the parking lot outside Connie's apartment building, but the trail vanished after that. The existence of Rikashi and his shipmates had not been released to the public, so a variety of cover stories was hastily prepared to justify the exhaustive search that ensued.

On the fourth day following her disappearance, Sarah was found wandering through a small park on the outskirts of Maclean. She was naked and disoriented but apparently uninjured. Connie rushed to the hospital room and was arguing with the security people when Kraft emerged from her sister's room and waved her through.

"She seems to be all right."

She brushed past him without a word. Sarah was awake, alert, and full of questions.

"What's going on, Connie? Who are these people? They act like police but they won't tell me what's going on."

"They're government investigators." Even under stress, Connie's training made her cautious. "How are you feeling? What happened?"

"I don't know. The last thing I remember was trying to decide what to do about supper, and then I had these dreams about . . . about the baby." She glanced away briefly, then back. "And then some people were putting me in an ambulance and they brought me here. But I feel fine, just confused is all."

They talked further until Connie felt reassured that Sarah was in no physical danger, then excused herself to find a doctor. She had little luck until Kraft intervened on her behalf.

"Your sister appears to be perfectly fine, Dr. Jensen. We won't know for certain until we have our test results back, but there's no indication of concussion, amnesia, or any physical trauma."

"But she can't remember anything that's happened for the past four days!"

The doctor shrugged. "Perhaps she was drugged. We'll know more when the tests are completed. But I assure you that they're both fine."

"Both?" Connie flashed an absurd scene, Rikashi in a hospital bed while a nurse took his pulse. Pulses, actually.

"Your sister *and* the baby," he answered testily.

"Baby? Dr. Weller, my sister isn't pregnant."

"I wasn't aware that your doctorate was in medicine, Dr. Jensen." Weller was openly sarcastic.

"It's not. It's in applied linguistics."

"Then perhaps you'll defer to a specialist. Your sister is very definitely pregnant, about thirty days along, I'd say."

Connie closed her eyes, opened them, spoke as calmly as she could manage. "Dr. Weller, I appreciate our relative positions here. But Sarah was severely injured two years ago. The doctors assured us that she was physically incapable of ever conceiving again. They were quite certain."

He paused only a second. "They were also quite wrong."

But even Dr. Weller expressed amazement when

Sarah's records were brought to the hospital by a government courier.

"There must be some mistake. Damage this extensive could not be repaired even surgically, let alone spontaneously. Are you absolutely certain that these are your sister's records?"

Two hours later, they found Rikashi. The alien was lying inside a culvert a quarter mile from where Sarah had been found. There were no apparent life signs and the body was taken away quickly and quietly.

Connie drove back to the compound, even though it was nearly midnight. The guard was used to people coming and going at odd hours and buzzed her through without comment. She went straight to her office, called up the transcript files, and began rereading every conversation she had conducted with Rikashi.

It was daylight when she finished and her brain was spinning with fatigue, and with alarm. She called the hospital, confirmed that there was no change in her sister's situation, and then drove home, fell asleep fully dressed, and didn't wake up until the middle of the afternoon. Awake once more she showered, checked with the hospital again, then called Colin Kraft.

"We need to talk," she said simply. "I'll meet you in your office."

"Are you telling me that the alien raped your sister?"

Connie shook her head. "The purpose of life is life.

I don't think Rikashi's species could even grasp the concept of forced procreation."

"But you think it impregnated your sister?"

"In some sense, yes. I think he realized how to repair the damage to her body, then somehow generated life. Whether there is any physical part of him in that life, I just don't know."

"The doctors didn't find anything unusual about the fetus."

"They weren't looking for anything either. But I don't know if there would be any discernible difference. Maybe there won't be until we realize it." She started to laugh, but it sounded hysterical and she stopped quickly.

Kraft remained thoughtful and she was glad he was taking this seriously. She doubted anyone else would. "For the sake of argument, let's say I accept that Rikashi and his kind can alter reality simply by believing they can do it."

"By realizing they can do it," she corrected.

"Whatever. Even if that's possible, humans don't have that ability. And Rikashi is dead."

"Is he?"

Kraft stared at her blankly.

"Life's changes never end," she quoted. "Rikashi's people believe in personal immortality."

"So do Baptists. What's the relevance?"

"I don't think they're as connected to their bodies as we are. They have difficulty interpreting sensory input consistently. They smell sounds or taste colors, neurasthenia. And I found several references in the transcripts to events of which Rikashi could have no direct knowledge."

"Telepathy?"

"I don't think so. I believe that their consciousness is linked to their physical location, but not limited to it."

"I see. Then you think that . . ." His face twisted into a grimace of distaste.

"No, not think, realize. I realize that Rikashi is still alive, and he's going to be my nephew."

A RUSTLE OF OWLS' WINGS

Thomas Smith

I HEAR THEM MOSTLY AT NIGHT. MOSTLY WHEN I sleep.

Sleeping.

Waking.

Sometimes I'm not sure which is which.

But I know I hear them.

The owls.

I hear them mostly at night.

I first heard them when I was a child. I dreamed about the owls. The owls with the big eyes. Staring. Probing. Watching me. Evaluating. Questioning. Talking without making a sound. Never a sound.

I remember how I used to sit in the dark, afraid to go to sleep. That's when I would hear them. Them and their rustling blue-gray wings. They were all blue gray. The owls who spoke without speaking.

I remember I used to sit in the dark and wait for

the sunlight. I prayed for the sunlight, but there was only darkness. Always too much darkness, and the big-eyed, soundless owls.

They asked me questions. Big questions. Questions I didn't understand then and don't fully understand now. Questions about where I came from and how I got here. I'm from here and I've always been here. I don't understand what they mean.

I've always been here.

And the owls have always been here. They have sailed the silver-black skies as long as there has been a sky to sail. Theirs is the whole universe, and they take wing at will and span time and space.

They say they are somewhat like us.

But they don't understand.

The first time I saw the owls clearly I was six. I had caught glimpses of them, seen them through the haze before that, but the Christmas I was six was the first time I really saw them.

We were at my grandma's house, had spent Christmas eve there; and though I loved Grandma Templeton better than almost anybody in the world, I couldn't help wondering how Santa Claus would ever find me. I hadn't told him in my letter that I was going to be gone. And once I realized my mistake I was afraid he would either leave all my toys at our house (and I would have to wait three days to see them), or find no one at home and just take them all back to the North Pole until next year.

But Mama said he would be able to find me. Santa has ways, she said. He always knows how to find you, wherever you are.

Somehow that thought didn't comfort me.

But Christmas eve turned into Christmas day, and he did indeed find me. Then Christmas day turned into Christmas night. And the house, so recently filled with light and the sound of carols, the smell of cider and evergreen boughs, turned dark and still and cold.

And they found me. They have their ways.

At first I sensed them more than saw them. I was asleep in the attic room of Grandma Templeton's big Victorian house. Over the years that huge room had been the lookout tower of a great castle, a rocket to the moon, Superman's fortress of solitude, and the site of a hundred other little boy fantasies. But that night those fantasies were lost forever. That night I felt something that shouldn't have been there—something that shouldn't be period—and shuddered myself awake from a sound sleep.

I rubbed my eyes and looked around the room. The forms around me took vague shape in the dim light of the moon. I saw the rocking chair in one corner and the faint image of the small Christmas tree against the far wall. I saw the dresser and the toy box, right where they had been for years. Everything exactly as it should be, exactly as it had always been, but nothing was right. The night was wrong. The lights were wrong. The light of the moon and the dust motes that swam down it's lunar stream was wrong.

As I lay there listening with every nerve in my body wide open to the slightest sound, straining to catch even the most minute change in the air, the chair in the corner started to rock. Slowly at first, then faster. Back and forth and back and forth. *Creee, thumpa. Creee, thumpa.* Faster and faster and back and forth until I knew it just had to tumble over and slide across the room. And all the time the chair—possessed with a manic life of its own—was rocking, the lights on the tree began to glow. Not all at once, but gradually. Like some unseen hand was slowly turning up a rheostat.

Without warning, the electric train began to travel around the base of the Christmas tree. Smoke poured from the stack, the headlight flashed, pistons advanced and retreated while the wheels clattered on the track at breakneck speed. *Clackity, clackity, clackity, clack, clack. Clackity, clackity, clackity, clack, clack.* Train and tree, carefully unplugged hours before, glowed and clattered while the rocker in the corner continued it's frenzied dance.

I wanted scream. To call out for help. But I couldn't. I couldn't speak. I couldn't move. I could only watch in a combination of mute fascination and abject terror as the other occupants of the room, inanimate until a moment earlier, mutinied against the laws of science and sense.

Clackity, clackity, clackity, clack, clack. Creee, thumpa. Creee, thumpa. Clackity, clackity, clackity, thumpa. Clackity, clackity, creee, thumpa.

I wondered why nobody heard. Wondered why my rescuers weren't already running up the stairs, rushing to pull me from the confines of my animated prison and rush me to safety. I looked down and willed my legs to move, to kick away the covers and carry me to safety, but they wouldn't move. They were as useless as if I had been paralyzed since birth.

My chest and throat burned with the effort of trying to make myself heard. A great internal pressure pushed against my rib cage, and I felt my lungs would burst any second.

You have nothing to fear from us.

The voice came from all around me.

You are safe.

More a thought than an actual voice. I didn't hear it so much as I was aware of it. Like someone else was thinking my thoughts for me. I tried my legs again without success.

Why do you struggle?

Even then the grand absurdity of the question was laughable, not that I felt the least bit like laughing then, or now. How could they not know I was terrified? Couldn't they understand I was just a little boy? And even though I tried to make the questions come out, tried to make them go away, the sensual onslaught continued.

The questions continued as did the reassurances. But I didn't want reassurance. I wanted them out of my room and out of my head. I wanted to wake up and find the train still, the tree dark, and the rocker sitting quietly in its place. But the train still whizzed around the track, teetering and smoking on every curve, the tree flashed in time to the thrumming of the train, and the already frenzied chair had increased its tempo.

Then, as quickly as it started, it stopped. Train, chair, and tree all ceased their macabre rondelet and went back to their previous inanimate existence as if nothing out of the ordinary had happened. In less than an instant they went from whirling dervish to deadly still.

Why are you afraid?

The large black eyes of the one speaking—I don't know how I knew that was the one, I just knew—were the last thing I saw before I passed out. The pressure in my lungs and the pressure in my mind needed a safety valve and unconsciousness was blissful release.

The rest of my memory of that night comes in bits and pieces. Flashes of coherence in the midst of insanity. I can remember a large gray room with a table or stretcher or some such thing in the middle of it. The owls were all standing around the table. Standing and staring. Watching. And the walls; the walls seemed to be moving in and out ever so slightly. I felt like I was inside something alive. Something breathing. In and out. In and out. Rippling and flexing. In and out.

All the while there were voices. The whole time I drifted between consciousness and oblivion, there were the constant voices. Voices that made no sound.

What are you?

. . . walls moving . . . breathing.

We must see . . .

eyes . . .

is in place and intact . . .

voices with no sound. pain. i need . . .

It is time to return . . .

The next morning found me in bed, Roy Rogers pajamas and bed covers rumpled, but no more than usual. I didn't remember anything beyond the time I first crawled into bed. I was nauseous until about noon and didn't have much to say—too much excitement had been Grandma Templeton's diagnosis—but there was no memory of anything other than going to sleep. Mama and Daddy packed up the car, and I packed up my memories. Buried them deep.

Thirty years deep.

I know I have seen the owls since then. I remember bits and pieces. I remember seeing the lights. And though I've never been to Texas, I can tell you what the Corpus Christie skyline looks like reflected in the water.

I remember vast expanses of black dotted with silver-white light.

I've been studying the owls. Learning what I can without having too many people look at me like I have a third eye.

I used to be afraid of the owls. Afraid of what they might do to me . . .

the pain

Afraid of what they have to say. But I'm not so afraid any more. Not so much. Because I've found others like me. Others who have seen things. Others who have feelings they can't explain and time for which they can't account. They haven't all seen owls—some can't remember just what it was they have seen—but they remember the eyes.

And together we remember bits and pieces. Some have seen the room with the table, and some have seen other things.

But we all remember the eyes.

And we all remember what it was like trying to explain to everybody we care about that our lives didn't seem to be our own anymore. We remember the eyes of our wives and husbands; the faces of our children. That's another memory we'd like to forget.

But even those things don't seem so important any

more. Not now. Because for some reason the memories of the owls have been coming in larger bits and pieces. And when I wake up fast enough, or write my thoughts down quick enough, I can make out more of what the owls were saying. Are saying. Not all of it, but more than before.

I've always been here. And they've always been here. The owls with the big black eyes. Eyes that watch and probe. Eyes as black as a bottomless pit.

But I've started to remember. And I've seen their pitch-black eyes up close. They're empty, haunting eyes. Empty, but not vacant. Not by a long shot. The owls know things. There is the wisdom of the ages in those eyes.

They have always been here. They have always been everywhere. This universe is their domain.

Every universe is their domain.

And they are coming back. Soon. I don't know how I know, but I know it as sure as I know my own name. And this time when they come, I am going to remember it all. The sights, the sounds, the smells. I'm going to remember every last detail.

They have been back many times, but I wasn't ready. They said so. They told me in my head and in my heart. But this time I am ready.

And I know they're coming back.

The sun is setting. Night is falling. And before long, they'll come for me. The blue-gray owls who speak without speaking.

I am going to sail the boundless reaches of time and space. The universe will be mine.

And just before we make the last transition and I stand poised on the edge of infinity, I am going to look back on who and what I was before the owls came. I am going to watch as the memory fades into the distance, and listen with a new understanding. And I am going to sail the silver-black sky as long as there is a sky to sail.

I will not be back.

FIREFLIES

P. D. Cacek

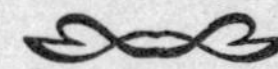

EMMA SLUMPED DEEPER IN THE CHAIR AND STARED AT her folded hands. Because it was better than watching the fat gray squirrels hopping through the late afternoon sunlight at the edge of the woods and remembering what it felt like—the still warm grass springy beneath her bare feet—to run after them.

Much better than remembering what it felt like to run.

What it felt like to *move* . . . by herself . . . without anyone's help.

Now that she couldn't.

Would never again.

Something hot and itchy tickled the corners of Emma's eyes, but she only clasped her hands tighter together until her fingers hurt. She could feel *that*, all right. Because she was still Emma from the waist up. Still Emma.

At least partways.

Wiggling her shoulders, she sensed the part she could still feel slip farther down . . . and watched the part she couldn't bend at the knees. It was funny—kinda—to watch the knees she couldn't feel anymore poke out from under the bright yellow blanket her mom always put over them. To keep them from burning, she said. But Emma knew better.

There was a Band-Aid on the right knee—the stupid Muppet kind they stick on babies. One of the nurses had put it there the morning Emma left the hospital. To make her smile. Like it was a joke.

Like she really would get better and not have to be crippled anymore.

Emma hated being crippled. *Hated* it. She even hated the word. Crippled. Cripple. It sounded like *ripple*. Like the icky *strawberry-cheesecake ripple* ice-cream her grandma always brought with her when she came to visit. Icky, yucky stuff!

Except Grandma wouldn't be coming to visit anymore. Couldn't. Because she died in the same accident that made Emma crippled.

Forever.

Emma heard the doctor telling her parents that at the hospital, whisper-whispering out in the hall while the nurse put the stupid baby Band-Aid on her knee to make her smile. "I'm so very sorry," Emma heard him say while her mom cried into the bunched-up tissues Daddy had got from the bathroom in her room, "but she's young. You'll be surprised at how well she'll adapt."

Adapt, adapt, a-snap . . . like what her back had

done when Grandma's car skidded sideways on a patch of gravel and hit that tree. *Snap* like a twig. Whisper-whisper like a little mouse. A little mouse in a little house. A little crippled mouse in a little crippled house dragging its little crippled legs behind it.

La, la.

Emma tossed the blanket over the bent knees and stupid baby Band-Aid she couldn't feel and thumped her fists against the wheelchair's shiny plastic armrests. And yelped. She kept forgetting how hard the armrests were.

"Honey? Are you okay?" her mom's voice called from inside the house. "What happened? Did you hurt yourself?"

Emma squeezed her eyes shut and held her breath. Maybe if she held it long enough she wouldn't be able to feel anything.

"Emma?"

Emma's cheeks pooched out like water balloons. She wrapped her fingers around the armrest, tight.

"Emma."

Colors began to swirl behind her puckered eyelids. Purple-yellow, red-green, blue-oran—

"Emma!"

The air popped out of Emma's mouth and she gasped. Turning her head, she saw her mom, still in the pink bathrobe she was wearing when she got Emma up that morning, staring at her from the other side of the patio's screen door. Looking scared. Taking a long drink from the tall Taco Bell cup she was always carrying around.

"Why didn't you answer me, Emmy?" her mom asked when she finally lowered the cup, using the baby name Emma had outgrown two years ago. "I thought you hurt yourself."

Emma shrugged and dropped her hands to her lap, crossing two fingers on her right hand and covering them with her left.

"There was a squirrel on the deck. I didn't want to . . . I wanted to see if it would come to me."

It was a fib, but she'd crossed her fingers so it didn't count. Maybe.

"Oh." Her mom smiled and took another long drink. "Want to come in now?"

Emma shook her head.

"Okay. But just a little while longer. The bugs'll be out soon."

Emma nodded. And watched her mom step backward into the purple shadows of the house. The sky was turning the same color. Emma looked up as she uncrossed her fingers. It *was* getting late. The edges around the clouds to the west (her daddy had showed her how to tell directions last summer—before the accident) were turning gold and coppery-pink, the lavender sky getting darker as she watched.

Becoming night.

Reaching down, Emma unhooked the latches on the big back wheels and rolled the chair almost to the edge of the deck.

It wasn't *fair!* Night was when the fireflies came out!

She shoulda been running through the woods right now, right this very minute, squishing up the soft ground between her toes and chasing them . . . right now . . . right this minute with a washed-out peanut butter jar in one hand and the coppery lid with its punched holes in the other. Just like last year. And the year before that. And all the other years Emma could remember since her daddy taught her how to catch fireflies.

Shoulda been.

But wasn't. Couldn't.

Besides, she thought, slipping down into the pillows her mom had lined the chair with, there weren't any more fireflies. Hadn't been since the lightning hit the woods not long after Emma had got back from the hospital. There hadn't even been a storm that night. All Emma could remember was a kind of high, windy kind of sound, getting louder and louder, until the flash of gold-blue-white light filled up her room.

And scared the fireflies away.

It wasn't fair.

Emma felt the tears sliding down her cheeks before she could reach up and swat them away, so she pretended she couldn't feel them. The same way she couldn't feel her legs.

Her daddy came home, car tires crunching gravel, while she was pretending. Brushing away the tears, Emma sat up and pretended to smile.

"I'm out here, Daddy," she shouted, pulling the chair back from the edge and turning it around. They didn't like her just sitting and staring at the woods—said it made her . . . *molasses* or something.

Her daddy's eyes (the same funny blue-green-gray as hers) got bigger and bigger when he came around the side of the house and saw her sitting there. And his mouth dropped open.

"What?" he gasped, throwing his suit jacket over one shoulder. The front of his shirt was all crumpled and wet, sticking to his skin so Emma could see the dark brown hair on his chest underneath. He had already taken off the bright red tie she had picked for him out of the dozen he brought into her room that morning. "Is the TV broken?"

"Oh, Daddy," she said, "I don't watch that much TV."

"Right," he said, trudging up the three steps to the deck as he wiped the shine off his face with the unbuttoned sleeve of his shirt, "and ninety-seven degrees isn't hot. So what brings you out into all this humid splendor when you could be inside an air-conditioned paradise watching *The Mighty Migraine Power Rangers* . . . or whatever they're called."

"Morphin," Emma corrected—just like she always did—and offered up her cheek for a kiss. Even his lips felt hot and sticky from the long drive home. "And they're only on on Fridays. Today's Tuesday, remember?"

"Ugh," he grunted as he squatted next to the chair, "don't remind me. Your mom know you're out here?"

Emma rolled her eyes and heard her daddy chuckle. "She knows."

Her daddy stood up and stretched, his forehead wrinkling suddenly. Groaning, he pressed one hand against his back.

"Well, as long as she knows." He yawned, still

rubbing his back. It took him a minute (or two) before he looked back down. "Tell you what, M&Ms, let me grab a quick shower and then I'll come back down and read to you until dinnerti—"

"Dinner in fifteen minutes," Emma's mom called through the screen door. "Why don't you bring Emma in and then take your shower? Hi."

"What a wonderful idea," he said, winking at Emma before turning toward the house, "why didn't *I* think of that. Hi, yerself, lady."

Emma felt the chair shudder when he grabbed the handles.

"Okay, pard, let's head 'em up 'n' move 'em out. Rawhide!" He always said that. Emma didn't know why.

"Can't I stay just a little bit longer?" she asked, her voice naturally going into a whine. "The 'squitos aren't even out yet."

Emma could almost hear the look that passed back and forth between her mom and daddy like a Ping-Pong ball. She turned her head and looked back at the woods.

"Just until the fireflies come out?" Oops, she forgot to cross her fingers. Emma clenched both hands. "Just 'till then, okay?"

She heard the screen door open. And swallowed. Maybe her mom knew about there not being anymore fireflies in the woods since the lightning.

Emma chewed a piece of summer-dried skin off her bottom lip and watched her mom tuck the blanket in around the legs she couldn't feel.

"Just until dinner's ready," she said, first ruffling,

then smoothing Emma's hair, "fireflies or no fireflies, got it?"

Emma looked up and smiled.

"Got it," she answered quickly, then watched her daddy and mom walk back into the house together; arms wrapped around each other's waists, like they were trying to hold each other up.

They didn't even look back when they closed the screen.

Pressing the sudden quiver out of her lips, Emma rolled the chair back to the edge of the deck and stared—*really, really hard*—not caring if she turned into a whole pile of molasses.

Not caring, but hoping she'd see a firefly even though that meant she'd have to come in. Because she missed them; almost as much as she missed running after them.

But the woods just kept getting darker—the spaces between the branches of the larch and beech and sycamores and maples and conifer pines (her daddy had taught her the names the same summer he taught her how to tell direction) just kept filling up with shadows.

Not fireflies.

When Emma was little (back when she didn't mind being called Emmy), she thought the flashing little lights were fairies and sprites, like the kinds in the stories her daddy read to her before she went to sleep. It'd been nice to think about them that way. But now she was a big girl and knew that they were only bugs with fires in their butts.

She giggled and covered her mouth so her parents

wouldn't hear. Then sighed and snuggled down against the back of the wheelchair. There was only a little bit of blue left in the sky above the woods when Emma looked up. Pretty soon her daddy would be back to push her inside for dinner . . . fireflies or no firef—

Something blinked.

In the woods directly in front of Emma, just to the left of the old maple tree that was always the first one to turn red in the fall . . . something *blinked*.

Grabbing the armrests, Emma pulled herself up and forward.

The something in the woods blinked again. And again. And *there* over by the larch Emma had tried to climb last spring, another blink. And there. And there . . . just below the first. And another.

Suddenly the whole woods behind her house was filled with tiny blinking lights that darted in and out and around the almost invisible trees, and left light trails floating in the air. Or seemed to.

The fireflies were back! But they were a different color than Emma remembered.

Before the lightning, they were a soft yellow-green color—like the flames of a hundred tiny birthday candles floating in the dark. But now they were all silvery-blue and so bright that they looked like little stars. One even glowed red . . .

The one that left the woods and flew slowly over the ferns and across the back lawn toward her; lifting and falling on the breeze like it was a tuft from a dandelion instead of a bug.

When it was only about a yard away from her, Emma made a small noise in the back of her throat and scooted the chair backward. It really *did* look like a dandelion tuft!

The other fireflies she caught, last summer when she could still run, looked just like big flies with glowing, yellow-green butts . . . this one . . .

Emma pulled hard on the wheels and crashed into the small redwood deck table she'd forgotten was there.

The bug hovered at the edge of the deck for a moment and looked at her. At least she thought it was looking at her . . . it *felt* like it was looking at her even though she couldn't really see it too well through the fuzzy red glow that surrounded it.

A second later it was moving again, getting closer. It stopped when it got above the blanket covering Emma's legs.

And smiled.

Now *that* was something she never saw a firefly do before.

Besides smiling, and having three teenie black eyes in the center of its "face" that blinked one at a time, this firefly didn't have any wings. At least none that Emma could see . . . and she really, really looked! Hard! Nope, no wings; just a bunch of glowing red spikes like a sea anem . . . anemen . . . anemenemi . . . *urchin* that swayed slowly back and forth and up and down.

Even its body was different. The fireflies last summer *looked* like flies. This one looked like a tiny person in a bright red suit.

"Did the lightning do that?" she asked it, whispering like she used to do in class so the teacher wouldn't hear.

The firefly got brighter; its smile widening until it stretched almost all the way across its face . . . *and then Emma felt it.*

The tingle.

In her legs.

Emma forgot all about the funny-looking bug, for a minute, and stared down at the rumpled blanket. The tingling got stronger, sliding up her thighs to where her legs met her body and down, over her knees, all the way to her toes!

"Ouch!" Emma's hand was halfway to the spot on her knee that was covered with the stupid baby Band-Aid before she stopped herself.

"I can feel my legs," she said, still whispering because she was afraid to talk any louder—afraid that she was really asleep and if she talked louder she'd wake herself up. "I'm not supposed to. How . . . ?"

The firefly smiled and held up one teenie-tiny hand. It had only two fingers on it, but that didn't matter, because now the tingling in Emma's legs was stronger . . . like it'd been her legs that had been asleep and now were full of pins and needles. It didn't hurt, not really, but Emma wiggled her toes anyway.

And giggled.

And suddenly was flying . . . *flying through a long, wide blackness filled with stars . . . millions of stars; tiny pinpricks* (tingles)*—all silvery white far off but changing as they sped past . . . changing into ribbons of blue to white to red. A million stars—a million ribbons of light that curved around them as they . . .*

They . . .

She turned without moving, her bright array of silver sensor/communication feelers swaying to the internal rhythm of the hive . . . she turned without moving and smiled at the others of her generational community, each smiling back in turn, each hovering within the beam of condensed light that served as transport.

Flying. Their thoughts feeding her, gliding to her through the bright white light that separated them from the cold blackness . . . the arms of her surrounding array curled inward, touching themselves to her mouth, to her mind, tasting, touching.

Tingling!

Emma jerked her head up and blinked. Did she fall asleep? She didn't think so . . . maybe . . . but the things she saw . . . the dreams about flying and the—

The big toe on her right foot suddenly cramped.

"Ouch!"

Ouch?

Leaning forward quickly, Emma pulled the blanket off her legs and wiggled the right little piggy that went to market. And watched the top of her sock move. Her mom always made her wear socks even though she couldn't feel it.

Hadn't been able to feel it!

Emma wiggled her left foot. Just to make sure. And giggled when the pins and needles prickled her.

Another tingle across the back of her neck made her look up. The firefly was hovering above her, waving its two-fingered little hand. She sat up. They were so close that Emma thought if she looked hard enough, she'd be able to see herself reflected three times in the bug's eyes. But she didn't even try to see, because the dreams of flying through the blue-white-red ribbons of stars in a bolt of lightning, and being able to taste feeling and moving . . . moving faster than she could have ever run before, filled the empty place in the pit of her stomach. Filled it and kept filling it until Emma stood up and took a step . . .

"Hey, M&Ms," somebody's voice called from inside the house, "ready to strap on the ol' feedbag?"

The firefly stopped smiling and darted back to the woods, taking the pictures and the feeling in her legs with it. Emma pitched forward, crashing face-first into the deck.

"Ohmy*god!* Emmy!"

Emma didn't care that he forgot and called her by her baby name, didn't even care that she'd fallen—not really—but it scared her because she couldn't feel her legs. Again.

She was sobbing loudly by the time her daddy got to her. His hands were warm and soft when he picked her up, his arms strong as they went around her. Emma grabbed the front of his T-shirt and buried her face in it.

"Oh, God, honey . . . are you all right? What happened?" His arms got tighter when she didn't answer. "Did you fall out?"

Emma nodded, wiping a sniffle off on her arm. It was easier than trying to tell her daddy about . . . what happened, because he would have said that was impossible, that she had fallen asleep or was telling a fib or *something.*

"I was—I was watching the fireflies and I just kinda . . ." She shrugged and felt his warm arm tighten around her. "Do you see them, Daddy? The fireflies?"

Emma didn't look until he nodded. "Yeah. Wow, look at 'em all. We got a good crop this year, all right."

So she looked and watched them dart in and out and around the dark branches—tiny silver lights and one red one—and knew she hadn't been sleeping or *something.*

"Okay, kiddo," he said, giving her one more hug before setting her back into the chair and stepping behind it, "time to come in, a deal's a deal, remember."

"I remember," she said but watched the fireflies until her daddy pushed her into the house and closed the screen door.

"Mum," Emma said around the mouthful of macaroni and cheese, "airs mu eanatutter jar?"

Her mother's fork with its speared piece of melon, stopped and hovered above her bowl—the same way the red firefly had hovered above Emma's legs.

"What?" her mother asked.

Emma swallowed. "My *peanut* butter jar. Do you know where it is?"

"It's in the cabinet in the kitchen," her mother said, quickly stuffing the melon piece into her mouth before setting the fork on the watermelon-shaped placemat and pushing her chair back from the table. "Why, do you want a peanut butter sandwich instead? I can go make one."

"I thought you liked macaroni and cheese,

M&Ms," her daddy said, looking straight across the table at her. "Don't you feel well?"

"Why wouldn't she feel well?" her mom asked, her voice suddenly all high and worried sounding. "Don't you feel well, Emmy?"

Emma scooped a giant-sized spoonful of macaroni into her mouth. And nodded. It took her longer than she thought before she was able to chew the glob into swallowable chunks.

"No," she said when she finally could, "the peanut butter jar with the punched out lid. For fireflies."

"Oh." Her mom looked calmer. A little. "Why do you want it?"

"I just told you, Mom . . . for the fireflies."

Emma sighed and pretended not to notice the *look* that passed back and forth between her mom and daddy like a Ping-Pong ball. It was a little game they had started playing since the accident: who was going to remind Emma about something she already knew.

Ping-pong.

Whack. Whack.

This time her daddy lost.

"But you know you can't chase fireflies, Ems," he said softly, trying to pass the *look* back to Emma's mom. But she was pretending not to notice either. "The ground's still pretty soggy from the rains we got last spring and, you know, those wheels aren't exactly the all-terrain kind . . ."

He stopped talking suddenly and picked up his glass of iced tea, finished half of it before setting it down.

"But I can get you a butterfly net and we can give it a try, if you like."

A butterfly net? For fireflies? Especially fireflies that could smile and make her legs tingle.

"No!" she shouted. "I need a peanut butter jar with the lid poked with holes just like last year. And you can't be there Daddy."

One of his eyebrows went up. "Oh? And why not?"

Because the firefly ran away when it saw you coming. "Because you're too *old* to catch fireflies."

Both her mom and daddy laughed.

"Okay, I'll give you that," he said, toasting Emma with the little bit of tea that was left in his glass. The ice tinkled like wind-chimes. "But I still don't think you're going to be able to handle that chair out in the—"

"I won't have to," Emma interrupted. She was getting awfully tired being told about things she *wasn't able to handle.* "All I have to do is sit real still and wait for them to fly over an' then I'll just catch 'em in the jar. So I really need my jar."

Her daddy was still smiling when he finished the tea and nodded.

"Okay, M&Ms, you win. I'll get you a jar."

"Tonight."

"I don't know if we still have one, Em—"

"Tonight."

"Em?"

"Please, Daddy? The fireflies are out there. You saw them."

Another look, but not the Ping-Pong one, crossed the table in front of Emma.

"Tonight," her daddy sighed. "Even if I have to finish off a whole jar of peanut butter."

He didn't have to eat a whole jar, just half of one. But he did moan with every mouthful . . . until Emma's mom sprinkled some chocolate chips in it. Then he got real quiet.

Emma watched him, smiling, rubbing her fingers lightly over the newly punched holes in the coppery lid. She'd made her daddy take the lid out to the garage to hammer in the holes—so the fireflies wouldn't see.

It still smelled like fresh roasted peanuts, even though her mom had washed it and popped out the waxy cardboard liner. It smelled good. It smelled like last summer . . . when she could still run.

Emma turned the lid over and ran her finger over the more jaggedy bumps. She used to be afraid, when she was little, that the fireflies she caught would hurt themselves if they flew up against one of the sharp inside-down holes, but her daddy had told her that any firefly *she* caught would be too smart to do that.

And none of them ever had.

Emma pressed her finger against one of the sharper ones until she forgot about last summer and running. A little.

Her daddy groaned suddenly and Emma looked up to see him holding his belly with one hand and the jar with the other. The jar was empty. Scraped clean.

Emma put the lid down in her lap and clapped her hands.

"You did it, Daddy!"

He looked at her and puffed out his cheeks. "What

I did was commit gastrointestinal suicide. God, it's like eating quick-drying cement!"

"Aw," Emma's mom said as she took the jar from him and carried it back to the sink, "poor baby. Nobody said you had to eat it all tonight."

"What? And let my daughter and the fireflies down?" He sat up straighter in his chair . . . for about a second before slumping back with another groan. "I'll never get that modeling job now."

Emma heard her mom laugh, but more importantly she heard the *sqweek swhish* of the dishtowel wiping the last of the water out of the clean peanut butter jar.

"Okay, here you go," her mom said, handing Emma the jar. It still felt warm from the hot water. "But I don't know about you going back out tonight. I mean there's probably a million mosquitoes by now and if you fell again . . ."

Emma gripped the jar and lid to the front of her T-shirt and glared at her daddy. *How* could *he? He told!*

Her daddy shrugged and rubbed his belly. Smiled with only half of his mouth. Emma hugged the jar tighter.

"I'll be okay," she said to her mom although she was still looking at her daddy. "I'm not gonna move . . . I gotta be real still so the fireflies'll come."

Emma heard the horrible "Well, I don't know . . ." and instantly changed her glare to a silent, round-eyed plea for help. This time her daddy didn't let her down.

"She'll be okay, hon," he said, groaning as he stood up and walked around to the back of Emma's chair. The chair creaked when he grabbed the handles and leaned on them. "I'll personally roll her out there and set the brakes. Heck, I'll even let the air out of the tires so she doesn't try to sneak off into the woods after those bugs."

"That's not funny, Ken—"

Emma didn't think so either, but she giggled anyway to show her daddy she forgave him for telling on her.

"Okay, kiddo, ready to pierce the nocturnal veil with its ravenous sanguineous warriors in glad hopes of luring a living speck of phosphorescent fire to its silicon prison?"

Emma looked back over her shoulder as he pushed her across the kitchen floor.

"Huh?"

"I asked if you were ready to sit outside in the dark and get eaten alive by mosquitoes while you wait for a firefly to come investigate your jar."

"Oh," she said. "Yeah!"

Emma heard her daddy mumble something about "blind faith" to her mom as they crossed into the family room. The patio lights were on and Emma could see moth shadows dance across the deck and railing. Beyond the railing it was all dark.

A little shiver tickled her back when her daddy wheeled her out to the middle of the deck and let go. She could only tell where the woods ended and the sky began by looking up and seeing the twinkling stars. There wasn't anything twinkling in the woods. No fireflies. Not yet. But she knew they were out there.

Somewhere deep inside Emma knew they were

waiting for her daddy to leave before showing themselves.

"Thanks, Daddy," she said, struggling to get the jar into her left hand and the lid into her right, hoping he'd take the *hint* in her voice.

He didn't. "You want me to stay out with you? Fight off any monsters that might be lurking about?"

Monsters? Boy, she wished he hadn't said that. "N-no thanks."

"Okay," he said. Emma could hear his bare feet whisper over the smooth wood as he walked back toward the house. "Holler if you need me. You want the light on or off?"

"O-off." The word kind of stuck in her throat. She swallowed. "How'm I gonna catch any fireflies if the light's on? And close the curtains too, okay?"

"You got it, squirt."

The porch lamp clicked off. There was only a little patch of light left, coming through the patio door, and she was sitting in it. Emma swallowed again.

"Just don't be too disappointed if none of the fireflies come out this far, okay, M&Ms?"

Emma nodded and heard the screen door slide shut. A moment later she heard the *swish, swish* of the curtain being pulled. A moment after that the darkness swept up over the railing and surrounded her. This was the scariest part—waiting for her eyes to get used to the dark so she could see—because *anything* could be already crawling out of the woods right now, right at this very moment, getting closer, and she wouldn't be able to see it.

. . . getting closer . . .

Emma almost called her daddy when she saw a tiny silver glow weaving in and out of the still almost invisible woods across from her. Almost before she could take another breath the woods were full of fireflies, just like before dinner. But all silver. Where was the red one?

As she leaned forward, squinting, trying to get a better look, the punched-out lid clinked against the side of the jar. It wasn't a very loud sound, but all the fireflies stopped—hanging in mid-air.

Although Emma couldn't see their tiny faces from where she was, she knew they were all staring at her.

"It's okay," she whispered, tucking the jar and lid down into the narrow space between the chair and her numb legs, "I won't hurt you."

Emma crossed the fingers holding the jar and held her breath. She could hear sounds from the house—fake laughter from the TV mixed with real laughter from her mom and daddy—and sounds from the woods—crickets and frogs down by the stream and . . . *ouch!* . . . the whine of mosquitoes.

But the fireflies still didn't move.

"Really," she promised, "it's okay."

They must have believed her because they started moving again, but not like the fireflies she remembered chasing *before* the lightning. They were lining up in two rows, just like she used to do at school when it was time to go home or go to an assembly or walk out in an orderly fashion during a fire drill . . . back when she *could* walk instead of having to be pushed by the teacher.

Emma shook the memory (and anger) away and

blinked her eyes. The two rows of silver fireflies were moving again, forming circles; one inside the other, each one going a different direction. She didn't know fireflies knew how to do that. Leaving the jar and lid where they were, Emma giggled and clapped her hands together. It was hard to do with crossed fingers but she managed.

Then, as she watched, the two spinning circles slowed and reformed back into two rows, leaving a narrow space between them for the red firefly. Emma giggled and clapped louder, her fingers uncrossing. She didn't bother to cross them again as the red firefly wove its way between the two silver rows, in-and-out-the-window, until it finally left the woods and flew straight across the dark lawn toward her.

"I knew you'd come," Emma whispered as it hovered over her lap. It was smiling. "I told my daddy all I'd have'ta do . . . I told my daddy you'd come."

Its smile widened and the black eyes blinked.

But Emma's legs still were numb.

She wiggled higher in the chair and the hole-punched lid *clunked* against something. Emma held her breath, but the red firefly didn't seem to have heard—it just kept smiling at her. She exhaled and smiled back.

Then she lowered her hands back to the lid and jar. *This was gonna be easy.* Fingers tightening, she looked past the red firefly to the hundreds of silver ones back in the woods. There were so many of them that she could probably catch four or five with a single scoop . . . if she were still able to run.

Emma turned back to the red firefly, blinked and

suddenly started dreaming, although she didn't remember falling asleep this time any more than she had the first time she dreamed about

Flying . . .

Hurrying along the pathways of the air with the others, tasting the excitement through her array as she followed the lineage of her generation back to the communal home hive.

The excitement—like the viscous nectar of the hatchling waters—coming from her and to her . . . condensing on the beam of light that streaked in jagged loops across the pale red sky.

They had come back, the others, from their journey through the darkness to an unknown light. They had come back to share the tastes and thoughts of their discovery.

She flew harder, opening her array to the minds of the assembled generations . . . the tiny sliver of hive brain that was hers alone seeing the beam of light that she and the others of her generation would travel in, through the darkness, past the blue-white-red ribbons to the waiting, tantalizing unknown light.

The sounds of the silence between the darkness humming, calling . . .

Buzzing!

Emma swatted at the mosquito buzzing around her ear and blinked as the dream vanished and the lid clunked against the chair again.

Her legs were tingling again.

She looked down at them, then back up at the firefly. Its smile looked different; wider, more open . . . like it was laughing. At her!

Emma picked up and jar and lid and moved them

to her lap. They felt cool where they touched the tingling bare skin of her thighs below the shorts. She forgot she hadn't been able to feel things like that either since the accident.

And it made her mad. First at herself because she'd forgotten and then at the firefly—for making her remember. For making her *feel.*

A tiny sliver of yellow light suddenly cut through the darkness next to her. Either her mom or daddy was peeking around the curtain, making sure she was still sitting there . . . making sure everything was okay. It made Emma even madder. The firefly turned toward the house, its tiny smile fading.

The pins and needles in Emma's legs and feet stung like a hundred-trillion bees when she stood up and swiped the jar and lid through the air.

"Emma!"

Her aim was a little off and the lid snapped off a dozen or so of the waving red threads before she was able to get it lined up and screwed down. The broken threads glowed for a moment, like dying sparklers on the Fourth of July, then went out. And when they did, Emma fell back into the chair, her butt smacking the canvas seat with a loud *thump.*

But she didn't feel it. Couldn't. Her legs were numb again.

"Emma?"

Although she heard her daddy calling, Emma pretended not to for a little longer and shook the jar like he showed her. It didn't hurt them, her daddy said, just made them forget which way was up so they couldn't escape.

She was panting when she finally stopped. The

firefly lay in a crumpled tangle in the bottom of the jar, its red glow faded almost to orange. It looked up at her through the curved glass wall of the jar and blinked its tiny black eyes.

It wasn't smiling anymore.

"I'm sorry," she whispered, first to the firefly in the jar then to the ones in the woods. "I really am."

Closing her eyes so she wouldn't be able to see the cold silvery light, Emma held the jar up over her head.

"Look, Daddy," she said softly, "I caught one."

When she didn't hear the soft scuff of her daddy's feet against the deck, Emma opened her eyes and glanced back over her shoulder. The look on his face made the jar in her hand suddenly feel heavier than it was. He was staring at her, at *her,* not the jar, his face all silvery with firefly light.

And it seemed to take a long time before he could get words to come out his mouth.

"Em . . . Emmy, were you . . . standing?"

Emma hugged the jar tight against her belly.

"Huh?"

But he was still standing there, holding on to the edge of the sliding screen door, and looking at her . . . hard—like when she couldn't get her fingers crossed in time and he knew it. Emma swallowed and licked her lips.

"Don't . . . don't you want to see the firefly I caught, Daddy? It, it came right up to the deck . . . just like I said it would."

Emma blinked when her daddy reached inside and turned the patio light on. He didn't seem to notice the light . . . or the fireflies in the woods beyond the deck . . . or even her. His eyes looked like they stopped seeing just before they got to her.

"Daddy?"

Then he shook his head and smiled. Maybe smiled. Emma wasn't sure it was a real smile, but she smiled back just in case it was.

"I must be tired," he said, mumbling, shaking his head before his eyes finally made it all the way out to her face. "For a minute there I thought . . ." Then he chuckled and Emma felt the pounding in her chest slow back down to a normal heartbeat. "Nuts. What? You said you actually caught a firefly? Gee, honey, that's great."

Emma watched her daddy take a step out onto the deck and suddenly slap the side of his head, near his ear. It was only then that she realized the mosquitos hadn't bothered her at all since she caught the red firefly.

Emma heard another hollow-sounding slap.

"C'mon, honey, we'd better get inside before the 'skeeters suck us dry."

Emma licked her lips as her daddy closed the distance between them and slowly held up the jar. She gave the firefly inside a quick glance before looking away . . . just long enough to see that it was still lying, crumpled, on the bottom of the jar and still looking up at her.

But it didn't look so bright anymore.

"Wanna see it, Daddy?" she asked, holding it higher.

Her daddy's look was even quicker than Emma's

had been. But he nodded at it and smiled. At least Emma thought he smiled, he could have been wrinkling up his face at another mosquito, because he shook his head and hunched his shoulders as he grabbed the handles on the back of her chair.

"You got a good one there, kiddo," he said as he pushed her back toward the house . . . and Emma suddenly remembered he'd said the same thing about the firefly she caught last summer (when she could still run) and the summer before that.

And the summer before that.

He didn't care. Hadn't cared.

Emma lowered the jar back to her lap and covered it with her hands. Held it close to her while her daddy pushed the chair through the family room and kitchen, down the hallway and past the living room to her room. Her "new" room on the first floor that used to be saved for when her grandma came to visit.

Hers now—and forever. Now that Grandma wouldn't be visiting anymore.

Emma tried not to think about it.

Tried not to think about *anything* as her daddy wheeled her into the room and started getting her ready for bed.

"Sure you don't want a story, M&Ms?" her daddy said, pushing her hair back off her forehead with one hand just like he always did before kissing her g'night. Just like always.

Except tonight he looked different. There were lines across his forehead that Emma didn't remember seeing before.

"Naw, that's okay," she said, sliding down, away

from his hand and watching (not feeling) her legs bend into weird shapes under the thin summer blankct. "I'm kinda tired. Catching fireflies is hard work."

"Yeah," her daddy said, nodding as he leaned down to kiss her. Emma felt the night stubble on his upper lip, all scratchy and prickly. Tingly. Pins and needles . . .

"—the matter, Emmy?"

Emma shook her head and blinked her daddy's face back. The lines on his forehead were deeper.

"Na-uh," she said, scrunching down. Away from the lines.

When she was tucked in, chin under the lemony-scented sheet fold, hair matting against the pillow, Emma turned to look out the window next to her bed. The window faced the woods, but all she could see were the sticky-out branches and the tops of the ferns, white with moonlight. She couldn't see any fireflies.

Not one. Outside.

In the glass she could see the dull red reflection from the peanut butter jar with the poked-out lid sitting on her desk.

Emma closed her eyes.

"Daddy? Could you put the firefly on the window-sill?"

She felt the bed shake when her daddy shifted his feet.

"It's fine where it is, honey. Now, get some sleep."

Emma opened her eyes when he stood up. "Please, Daddy?"

The light from her bedside lamp made his shadow

go all the way up the wall and on to the ceiling. When he shook his head he looked like a giant.

"I dunno, honey, you might turn over in your sleep and kick . . . knock it over and—" He shrugged and the giant filled the room.

"But I think it's hungry, Daddy," Emma said, remembering something he'd told her when she was still a baby. "You said fireflies glow because they eat moonlight. And the moon's still out, so . . ."

When Emma heard her daddy chuckle she knew she'd won.

"Okay, okay," he said, the giant shadow moving away, across the room. It looked less scary when it came back with the shadow jar in its hand. "Far be it from me to let a firefly miss its dinner. There. How's that?"

Emma sat up and nodded at the jar's placement—halfway between her head and the two lumpy mounds that were her feet.

"Thanks, Daddy," she said, lying back down . . . and throwing in a yawn for good measure. " 'Night."

" 'Night, Ems," he said, giving her a second kiss on top of her head, "sweet dreams."

"You too, Daddy," she answered and closed her eyes; turned over onto her side, hoping her bottom half had made the turn with her.

She didn't move from that position until after the room went dark and she heard her daddy's footsteps clump, clump, clump down the hallway all the way back to the family room. *Then* she sat up and found that her bottom half was still twisted more or less the other way. Most other nights that would have bothered her, but tonight she didn't care.

Tonight would be the last time she'd ever have to care about that, or being crippled, ever again.

Sitting up, Emma scooted herself down along the mattress (ignoring the way her legs bent all funny under the blanket) until she was even with the jar. The firefly looked asleep.

Picking the jar up with both hands, Emma shook it just hard enough to wake up the glowing red bug.

It opened two eyes, the third one stayed closed.

"Okay," she whispered to it through the holes in the lid, "I'm gonna open this but you gotta promise you won't fly away, okay?"

The firefly looked up and blinked. Emma took that as an "okay" and nodded.

The tips of her fingers were sweating as she opened the lid. She really didn't know what to expect—even though this firefly didn't look or act like *any* of the others she'd caught over the years, she couldn't be sure it would keep its promise. The dream/picture started the moment she lifted the lid off the jar.

Only this time she wasn't flying.

And there wasn't any tingling, pins and needles feeling in her legs.

This time she was

. . . *dying* . . .

Emma gasped, her heart beginning to pound in her chest, and tried, really tried, to blink herself awake. But she couldn't stop herself from dreaming anymore than she could stop herself from reaching into the jar and scooping the unmoving firefly into her hand. Another dozen red milkweed hairs broke off as she lifted it toward her face.

She didn't like touching bugs, always making her

daddy take out the firefly after it had gone dark and died in the jar . . . but this time it was different . . . this time she felt

. . . empty . . .

A million ribbons criss-crossing the darkness—blue-white-red—a million generational clusters to touch, feel, savor.

Only to come to this, separated from the others, taken alone.

Empty . . . emptied . . .

Dying in the darkness, far from the touch and feel of the others . . . the ribbon of light fading . . . emptying itself into the darkness—no sound, no touch, numb.

The light fading.

The light.

Emma curled her hand around the firefly as she squinted into the bright silver light that suddenly poured in through the window next to her. It was so bright she could barely see them, the silver fireflies, hovering just beyond the screen, pressed against it . . . hard to see, they were so bright.

So bright.

Emma felt something move against the inside of her palm and opened her hand. The firefly didn't move and it wasn't glowing anymore. Biting her lower lip, Emma poked at it with a finger.

Poked it harder.

Its body rolled over, the drooping milkweed hairs curling around it like a cocoon. It was dead. Emma had seen enough dead bugs to know what a dead one looked like.

"You can't be dead," she told it, closing her hand and shaking, just to make sure it hadn't fallen asleep.

She knew it wasn't asleep when she opened her hand.

"You *can't* be!" Emma yelled at it through the bright silver light. "You gotta wake up and make my legs tingle again. Please? Please!"

"Emmy?" Her daddy's voice echoed from down the hall. "What's the matter?"

Emma didn't answer. Closing the hand that held the dead firefly, she leaned forward and reached toward the window . . . felt the tingle the moment her knuckles brushed against the screen.

If she could catch one of the silver fireflies . . .

Emma reached for the screen's latch just as the door to her room opened, a wave of butter-colored light crashing against the silver.

"Ems? What the—"

The fireflies broke apart like a thousand shooting silver stars and darted back across the lawn, over the tops of the sleeping ferns, and through the wood's laced branches until they were lost in the darkness beyond the woods.

The sob broke from Emma's throat a moment before the tears came.

"Emmy? It's all right." And then her daddy was next to her; the bed shaking, tossing her into his arms. "What's the matter, baby? Did you have a nightma—Jesus!"

The bolt of lightning cracked the sky apart, a silver-white scar in the dark. Like the tiny scar on Emma's leg. The one she couldn't feel. Would *never* feel.

Emma pushed her face against her daddy's T-shirt and sobbed louder.

"Oh, honey, that's okay . . . it was only lightning.

Pretty close too, it sounded like." He patted her back, stroked her head. "It's okay, baby. The lightning won't hurt you . . . remember when lightning hit the woods a while back? Nothing happened, right? Oh, baby, what is it?"

Emma held out her hand and opened it, but she didn't look. Didn't want to see.

"The firefly's dead, Daddy."

Her daddy chuckled and Emma sobbed louder.

"Oh, baby, that's okay," he said. The bed shook again and Emma felt coolness against the wet on her cheeks when he turned and shook the dead firefly from her hand to his, "you can catch another one tomorrow night."

Emma shook her head as he got up and tossed the crumpled thing into her wastepaper basket.

"N-not like this one."

"Oh, sure you will, Em. Look, I'll even help. Tomorrow night, just you and me and the peanut butter jar. We'll get us a firefly that'll make this one look sick."

"But daddy, you don't underst—"

"Is everything all right in there?" her mother called—her voice sounding far away and angry.

Her daddy hunched up his shoulders and tiptoed quickly back to her.

"Scoot down, honey. There." His hands tucked her in. His lips touched her forehead. "Now, go back to sleep and dream about fireflies, okay? 'Night."

The butter-colored light went away.

Emma listened to the footsteps getting softer and softer until her own sniffling was all she could hear. The fireflies were gone, she knew that. The lightning had taken them away. There wouldn't be any to catch tomorrow or the night after that or the night after that.

Never.

Emma cried for a long time. But when she finally fell asleep she didn't dream.

A WORLD HUSHED BY SNOW

Juleen Brantingham

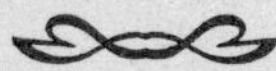

I WAS EIGHT YEARS OLD ON THAT SNOWY NIGHT. Eisenhower was president and aliens had come down from the stars to meet us but I was eight years old and the most important thing in the world was that there was two feet of snow on the ground.

A year and a half before I had moved with my parents to Ohio from Louisiana. I'd never seen snow in the south and the previous winter, our first in the north, had disappointed me. There had been too little snow, just a flurry now and then, scarcely enough to whiten the ground. This year would be different, according to the weatherman I listened to with an almost religious devotion. This year, he said, there wouldn't just be snow, there would be *snow!*

No one in my family looked forward to it more than I. Certainly not my soft-spoken mother, who endured exile with an air of martyrdom. Nor my father, a teacher, whose views on certain scientific subjects had led to his being fired from his last position. He lived and worked in a fog in those days, preoccupied with the aliens that had landed in Washington and what their presence might mean, particularly as regarded our relations with Russia.

Snow was predicted but had not yet fallen that evening. As I listened to the weather report before supper I was aware of the tension between my parents. Father was reading a newspaper report about the aliens and Mother was fretting out loud about Father's chances of finding a new position, perhaps in a private school in New Orleans.

"Let's see what develops in Washington before I send out any more letters," Father said finally, closing the newspaper and smoothing its pages.

For the rest of the evening, Mother's face wore the pinched look it got when she was angry beyond words but it wasn't until after I went to bed that their disagreement turned into a shouting match.

It must have been about 2:00 A.M. when I was jerked out of a sound sleep by raised voices from downstairs. The sound made my heart thump, made my stomach feel queasy. My parents *never* argued and *never* raised their voices. Something must be wrong, I thought. More wrong than I knew when I went to bed. Maybe the aliens had killed President Eisenhower. Maybe Mother was going to divorce Father.

Then I looked out the window. The aliens, the president, my parents, and all their concerns might have disappeared off the face of the earth for all I knew or cared. It was snowing! Fat white flakes were drifting down from the sky. There were little piles of snow in the angles of the crosspieces that held the window panes. I ran across the room and pushed the window open, stuck my head out and opened my mouth to let the flakes fall on my tongue. I can still remember that first taste, like electricity if you could taste just a drop of it.

The view of our front yard, the road, the field beyond was a magical sight. It wasn't snowflakes falling from the sky but flakes of light. The layer that blanketed the ground was as bright as the moon. In the clear patches between the clouds, stars burned like the diamond necklace my grandmother wore with her good black dress.

The world had gone still, as if it was holding its breath. Cold air tingled the inside of my nose.

Below, in the living room, my parents continued to shout. I cannot describe the way that made me feel—tormented, disbelieving, angry—none of those words quite encompasses the turmoil. But there was snow on the ground and snow still falling. It was as if I was in another world, a world where my parents didn't exist, a world hushed by snow.

Snow. The word sizzled in my blood and thickened the air in my lungs. I could not go back to bed and wait for morning like the well-behaved child everyone believed me to be. Suppose it all melted away before the sun came up! Thinking back on it now I suppose my urgency had more to do with the fears ignited by hearing my parents shouting at each other than it had with the snow itself. But I was eight years old and if my world was going to end with my parents divorcing or if aliens were going to blast the earth to pieces, I was determined not to miss my chance to play in the snow.

The coat closet was within sight of thc living room but it didn't take me long to solve that problem. I had plenty of shirts, sweaters, pants, and even an old pair of galoshes in the back of my closet. I could cram my feet into the floppy boots if I didn't bother with shoes. My hat and scarf were on the floor where I'd tossed them after coming home from school. A couple pairs of socks on my hands took the place of mittens.

Getting out of the house was easy. There was a back staircase that led to the kitchen. I was outside in scarcely more time than it takes to tell.

After closing the door, I tiptoed across the porch, avoiding the fan of light that spilled from the living room's rear window. Down in the yard my footsteps crunched, a mystifying and delightful sound. I had always thought of snow as being as light and soft as feathers. The flurries of the previous winter had done nothing to change my mind. I knelt and plunged my hands into a snowdrift, then tossed handfuls of it up into the air.

When I got to my feet it was only so I could topple backward and make a snow angel, a trick I had heard about in school. I must confess that I was not as detached from my parents' troubles as I pretended. In the split second before I fell back to make my angel I had the thought that it might make Mother smile to look out in the morning and see an angel beside the back steps.

I took giant steps to the far end of the yard. The house my father had rented for us was surrounded by farmland, except for a small stone house nestled on a narrow strip to the north, separated from our yard by a few rotting posts and strands of wire. Northwest, a mile away, was the railroad bridge that crossed the river. I was strictly forbidden ever to go near the railroad tracks or the river. Naturally I had explored both within a day of moving into the house.

But it was the stone house and its occupants, an old man and about a thousand cats, that drew me to the far end of the yard again and again. I had seen the man only once or twice—bearded, dirty, with red eyes—and spoken to him never, but he looked much more dangerous than a river or a railroad bridge and thus was the greater attraction.

That night there seemed to be candles burning behind the curtains that covered his windows. Judging from the shadows that flickered there, it looked as if his thousand cats were dancing madly. But silently. None of them came to peek out the window at me so after a while I gave up spying.

Kneeling with my back to one of the fence posts, I made cigarette-puffs of my breath and I curled my toes—now painfully cold with only a couple pairs of woolen socks and a thin layer of rubber to protect them. When I did that, the snow creaked. For sheer pleasure I toppled sideways, then rolled over on my back. It had stopped snowing and the fat-bottomed clouds had sailed away, leaving a sky so deep and dark and burning clear I felt as if I might fall into it, touching the stars with my soggy sock-mittens as I passed by.

I sat up and pushed the edges of my stocking cap up over my ears. I listened. Hard. I had never before and never since experienced such a great stillness. Listening hard is like staring hard: soon your straining senses create sounds or sights that are not real. For me it was a high-pitched metallic buzz that faded in and out.

I shook my head to dislodge the pain of that bone-aching buzz.

My next stop was the falling-down shed where Father kept the lawn rake he'd bought a month and a half ago to gather up the leaves from the cherry and pear trees in the back and the maple trees that lined the road in front. The roof of the shed had a hole in it. Father kept saying he was going to talk to the landlord about repairing it but he never did. He told me never to go inside because the roof might fall down.

I think I mentioned that people believed me to be a well-behaved child. I didn't say I was one.

The shed, too, was familiar territory. More than once I had scuffled through leaves and wind-blown trash to prowl among the stacks of rotting cardboard boxes lined up against the back wall or to climb the stagelike platform next to those boxes and recite poetry or have imaginary sword fights.

As I stood in the doorway I noticed a faint shadow. I turned to see the moon behind me, low in the sky. It looked as big as Mother's turkey platter.

I was all alone in the world, it felt like.

Then I heard a sound, a clinking rattle from the back of the shed. My insides turned as cold as the snow. The noise couldn't have been made by anyone who had a right to be in there.

Maybe it was the old man.

Or five hundred or so of his cats getting set to attack me.

Before my heartbeat slowed down there was another noise, a brushing sound, soft but heavy. A tramp, I thought. I wasn't entirely sure what a tramp was but my mother seemed dreadfully afraid of them. She thought rivers and railroads were the sort of places they would come from.

My mind raced, dreaming up more possibilities, most of them dangerous and all of them exciting. Minutes ticked by. The escaped bank robber/runaway circus elephant didn't seem to want to come out. Then I heard the noise again and the person who made it stepped into the doorway.

It was a kid.

The night was even more magical than I'd thought when I saw the snow. I might have created that kid myself out of loneliness and wishes. I didn't throw my arms around him and whoop with joy but to me a runaway circus elephant couldn't have been more exciting. There weren't any other kids out where we lived and the kids at school—well, in the fifties, in Ohio, my accent and the fact that my father was a teacher marked me as a target, not a possible friend.

But what was this kid doing out here, so far from town, at this time of night?

Being properly brought up, I introduced myself before I asked him. He didn't answer.

He—I've always assumed *he,* though I never found out for sure—he was dressed the same as I would have been if I'd managed to get to the coat closet. He had on a thick jacket that was a little too big, probably to allow for two or three sweaters underneath; besides the jacket he had on snow pants, boots, mittens, a scarf wrapped around the lower part of his face, with a knit cap pulled down over his eyebrows. He looked like a fat doll or a boy-shaped sausage, the same as I would have looked in the outfit my mother considered suitable for the arctic chill of Ohio.

"What's the matter with you? Cat got your tongue?"

He raised a hand, slowly, as if he wasn't sure of the gesture.

Annoyed, I squatted down, scooped up some snow, and made the first snowball of my life. It wasn't a very good one. When it hit the kid, smack in the middle of his overstuffed jacket, it split apart so fast he probably hadn't felt it.

For a second he didn't move. Then he bent his head to look at the dusting of snow on his jacket.

From the old man's house came a sudden yowling, as if a dozen cats had, all at the same time, got their tails caught under the rocker of his chair. I jumped about six feet but I never took my eyes off the kid.

Still with his head bent, he kept leaning over like he was going to topple head first onto the ground. Then he dropped his arms and scooped up a double handful of snow, packed it a bit, and tossed it at me. His snowball was worse than mine. It fell apart in midair.

"You do it like this," I said in what I am sure was a disgusting tone of superiority. I showed him how I thought it should be done. When I had it packed hard enough to suit me, I threw it at a fence post.

It struck the post and made a satisfying *thwack*.

I turned, grinning. The other kid was making a snowball the way I'd showed him.

Together we pounded the tar out of that fence post.

My memories of the next hour are hazy. The kid and I raced around, threw snowballs, climbed the pear tree and shook branches to make snow shower down, made snow angels and a lopsided snowman. All in silence. Well, I laughed a couple of times but stifled the sound, aware of Mother's keen hearing. The kid never made a sound but I could tell he was having fun, too.

That came to an end shortly after the kid fell down and I fell on top, straddled him, and washed his face with snow. I didn't choke or stare—my mother's child could never be so rude—but his was not a human face.

The cats yowled again.

Red light washed over the snow.

I scrambled to my feet, trying to see where it was coming from. I think the other kid got up then too but the light and the rising yowl of the cats, accompanied by a metallic buzz, confused me. Turning away, I looked at the house. The commotion and light from a direction that should have been dark and silent at this time of night should have brought my parents racing to the window but there was no sign of them, nobody called my name.

I suspect now that the lights and sound were contained somehow, as if the kid and I had been playing in some sort of protective cell.

I turned back to see if I could make out the other kid, if he was all right. Lights came down all around us, green and purple, blue and pink, like Christmas tree lights but with nothing that I could see connecting them. The kid—I could make out his silhouette against the lights—was floating two feet off the ground.

He beckoned to me.

It seemed perfectly natural. He had played in my yard. Now he was inviting me to play in his.

I didn't speak, but inwardly, feeling like it was Christmas morning, I said yes. When I did, my body started to rise.

I had risen as high as the second story of our house when I saw the hall light come on and realized my parents were on their way to bed. The last thing my mother did at night was to look in on me. She would see my empty bed. I knew how she would feel when she realized I wasn't in the house.

My body sank back to earth.

The lights had disappeared by the time I reached the porch and the cats' yowling had almost faded away. All that was left was the metallic buzz, which I still sometimes feel and hear at odd times and in odd places.

I managed to get into the house about two minutes after Mother saw my empty bed. Father gave me a paddling anyway.

The next spring Father was offered a position at a private school in Baton Rouge. We moved back home and I've never left. Sometimes I miss the snow. Or maybe it's not the snow but rather that special feeling you get sometimes on a snowy night when everything is hushed and still and so strange that it might be some world other than earth.

If you were alive during the time Eisenhower was president you don't remember anything about aliens landing on the lawn of the White House. If you study the history books or look up the back issues of those newspapers and magazines my father studied so closely, you won't find anything about the incident.

There's one person who might know something, if you can find him. A couple days after that snowy night I was playing in the back yard when I saw the old man come out of his house. He stopped to look at me. His eyes were very red.

"For your own good, don't talk about what happened. Ever." Then he walked on.

Mother said he moved out of the stone house that winter but I don't remember seeing a moving van or even a car.

Years later Father told me that when Mother saw my empty bed she screamed, "My baby's been kidnapped by aliens!"

We had a good laugh about that.

AFTER WELLES

Michael Scott Bricker

THE ODD HAD BECOME COMMONPLACE, THE ORDINARY, all too rare. While driving home through downtown Grover's Mill, New Jersey, I was slowed by a passing military convoy, and was reminded of the war in Europe. Jeeps and big, heavy trucks secreted what I assumed to be Martian goods along the eastern road. Spindly mechanical legs, blackened, muddied, poked out from under a massive tarp on one of the larger trucks, and I wondered if another ruined Martian machine had been uncovered. Somewhere under that tarp was a heat ray, I assumed, and I imagined scientists and military men examining their find in locked rooms, drawing diagrams, blueprints, building prototype machines, Martian weapons, splashed with air force insignia. I imagined U.S. machines crawling into Europe, going up against Nazi war machines, cities obliterated in the flash of a heat ray.

The United States *would* become involved, it was inevitable, and in human hands, the new weapons could finish the mission that the Martians had failed to complete. By handing us the tools of our own destruction, I thought, the Martians might have won, after all.

I feared that Ruthie would find a gift of Martian origin to be distasteful, or worse, offensive. And yet . . . it was a handmade silver brooch, a product of black market artisans, more beautiful than any I had ever seen. Spun silver, little intertwined bows fashioned into the image of a rose, and at the center, a polished Martian mirror. I rubbed my thumb across the surface of the mirror and thought of the girl who had sold it to me, her gentle face (so beautiful, I imagined, before a heat ray had bubbled her skin), and I wondered why she would sell artifacts which would certainly hold painful memories. The centerpiece of the brooch, that fantastic, reflective mirror, had been crafted from a shattered heat ray assembly, taken from a Martian Cylinder which had been discovered only a month ago by a worker with the New Works Progress Administration. That was what she told me, and I had no reason to doubt her, because as I held the brooch in the sunlight, rotated it in my palm, the mirror changed color, red then yellow then blue, and I felt that nothing of earthly origins could be so beautiful, so frightening.

They had nearly destroyed us all.

The New Jersey State Militia was out in force, uniformed men wandering along crumbling walks, stopping people, searching packages, and as I drove slowly down Main Street, I took the brooch from my coat pocket, reached down, dropped it beneath the seat. Grover's Mill was slowly coming back to life. A new building was going up where the old Owl Drugs had been, a cold, formidable structure in brick and steel. All of the new buildings were like that, built for strength and utility, void of ornament, as if to show the world, the *universe,* that we were not to be provoked. I missed Owl Drugs. It had been in an old brownstone with apartments above, and I would have lunch there almost every day. I had eaten lunch there on the afternoon of October 30, 1939. Hours later, the first cylinder had impacted.

The militia was stopping automobiles ahead, asking questions. I thought about Ruthie, hoped that she would still be waiting for me if I was late. It took twenty minutes for my Plymouth to make it to the front of the line, and as it did, I remembered the photograph on the seat next to me.

"Where are you coming from?" The uniformed man leaned over, reached in, put his hand over the steering wheel.

If he saw the photograph, what would he do? He might search the automobile, find the brooch, fine me or put me in jail for possessing Martian goods. *But if he saw the photograph, what would he do?*

"What's wrong? Didn't mean to startle you."

I was staring at the photograph, hadn't realized it until the man spoke. "Sorry. On my way out of town. Business—"

"You all right?"

I turned, looked at the uniformed man, was relieved

to find that I knew him. His name was Jim Breckenridge, and he used to live in Morristown before the invasion. "Jim, it *is* you, isn't it?"

"Sure. Haven't seen you in some time." He paused. "I've stayed away from New Jersey during the last year. Now I'm in the militia. Too much free time. Had to do *something.*"

Although it had only been a year since I had last seen Jim and his wife, he looked years older, and he carried himself awkwardly. I wondered what could have happened to change him so, and then I remembered the Morristown Cylinder. It had given birth to three of the most destructive Martian Crawlers of the invasion. After choking the countryside within a fog of poisonous black smoke, the machines had joined three more then moved toward New York City. Jim, who had been away on business at the time, lived through the invasion. His wife and two children had not.

Jim paused, stared at the seat next to me. I knew he had seen the photograph, watched his face grow pale. He took his hand from the wheel, backed up, said, "Move along."

I sensed no emotion in his voice, and it was obvious that I was no longer welcome, an invader like those leathery creatures which had taken his family. As I drove off, I wondered why Jim hadn't taken me into custody, and I imagined that he no longer had any fight left, that the Martians had taken his spirit as well. The photograph kept me company as I left the repopulated main drag of Grover's Mill behind and headed for the ruins of the Wilmot farm. I held the photograph as I drove, stared at the beautiful image of Ruthie and I holding hands, and I wandered from the dirt road now and then as I thought about how severely the local laws might punish a white man like myself who had been photographed while holding hands with a Negro woman.

Ruthie waited at the Wilmot farm. I found her standing at the edge of the crater where the first cylinder had impacted. When I touched her shoulders, she barely reacted. "All dead."

"What?"

She turned, embraced me. "All dead."

"I know." *Who were dead?* I wondered. Certainly not the Martians. We were still being watched, *scrutinized.* That was what journalists like Edward R. Murrow and Orson Welles had reported, and even the noted astronomer Professor Pearson reasoned that one day the Martians would learn to combat the earthly disease bacteria which had ended their lives, and they would try again.

The roof of the farmhouse had burned and fallen in, and not far away, blackened wood littered the ground where a heat ray had struck the silo. I wondered why the Wilmot Farm had not burned to the ground, and I remembered hearing that Martian heat rays burned only those areas which they were focused upon, that they rarely ignited larger fires. Their destruction was very precise and complete, just as the Martian invasion might have been had the bacteria not stopped them.

Ruthie gently pushed me away and said "Someone might come. They might see us."

"Nobody comes here anymore," I said, and I

wondered how much longer that would be true. The first Martian machine had risen out of this crater, over the rim where Ruthie and I stood, and its heat ray had burned forty people in a matter of seconds. It took several days to recover the bodies.

"There are ghosts here." Ruthie held my hand and guided me towards the farmhouse. "They talk to me sometimes."

I picked up a blackened stake from the weed-choked garden and knocked off shards of glass from the frame of a broken window. We crawled in and found ourselves in the Wilmots' kitchen. I was surprised by how modern the kitchen looked, not at all like what one might expect from the owners of a small farm. Along the wall, pots, pans, and burnt timbers were scattered on the floor near a new white enameled kerosene range and a porcelain cabinet. I saw an electric refrigerator near the opposite wall, and wondered how the Wilmots had afforded it. Electric refrigerators cost at least one hundred dollars, while an icebox could be had for less than twenty. I felt a chill; the touch of Ruthie's ghosts, of autumn. It was two days until Halloween, and tomorrow would be the first anniversary of the invasion.

I hoped that the Wilmots had enjoyed their farm before the Martians had taken their lives. Bob Wilmot, his wife, their two children; all killed in one, terrible blast of a heat ray.

"I've brought you something," I said, then reached into my coat pocket and handed the brooch to Ruthie. I gently closed her fingers around it. "A year. Nearly a year."

"Our first anniversary." Ruthie smiled, opened her hand, and sunlight reflected from the mirror into her deep brown eyes, against her smooth, dark skin. She was so young, so beautiful, and at twenty-six, she reminded me of a girl of eighteen. Again I thought of the girl who had sold the brooch to me, of how a heat ray had disfigured her so, of how grateful I was that Ruthie had escaped a similar fate. "I'm sorry," I said. "I didn't know what to get for you. It's a terrible gift. *I'm sorry.*" I felt foolish for giving the brooch to Ruthie. It was irresponsible, even cruel. If the militia found her with it, she would be arrested.

"It's beautiful," Ruthie said. "Don't worry. I'll be fine."

"Will you?"

She hugged me, laughed uncomfortably. I could feel tremors moving throughout her body. "It's not nearly as bad anymore. It's been weeks since anyone has thrown rocks. Maybe they've decided that I'm not a Martian after all."

"It's stupid, ridiculous." I said. Ruthie looked beautiful and I told her so, told her that people who refused to acknowledge her beauty were blinded by ignorance. I embraced her, wrapped her in my pale arms, and then I saw a Forager peeking through the window.

He was perhaps fifteen years old, and he had wild, matted hair and a feral look about him. Like many Foragers, he had painted his face in the Martian style, had streaked soot from the edges of his lips so that it appeared as if his mouth formed an inverse V. I remembered the reporter's radio broadcast during the evening of the invasion, as he stood on the edge of the Wilmot Crater, as a Martian emerged from that first cylinder. It was horrible, he had said, "the most terrifying thing he had ever witnessed. Tentacles, wet leather, V-shaped mouth dripping with saliva, large as a bear."

"Don't worry," I said. "Foragers work on the wrong side of the law. He won't tell anyone." I had no sympathy for Foragers, and had Ruthie not been with me, I might have gone after him, turned him in. It was rumored that the Nazis had harnessed heat ray technology, and Foragers were precisely the sort who were responsible. They were scavengers of the worst sort, selling Martian artifacts to whoever would pay, no questions asked. The U.S. government still considered Grover's Mill to be an important strategic area, and weird bits of Martian machinery were still being found in abandoned fields or on the bottom of shallow lakes. It was technology which we wanted to keep in the United States, technology which could win a war, or prolong one.

"I worry about you. You're not safe with me." Ruthie paused, and after an awkward silence she said "You should find a white woman. It would better for you."

Her comment angered me, and I pulled back. "I don't care what color you are, white, yellow, green . . . I really don't think about that sort of thing. I'm not some backward paranoid idiot . . ."

Ruthie began to cry, and I held her close, hated myself for my outburst.

"I'm sorry," I said. Ever since the invasion, racism

had been on the rise. This was particularly true in Grover's Mill. Ignorant locals had accused a Negro family of helping the Martians, had developed the moronic theory that Negroes had Martian blood. I watched as friends were jailed on trumped up charges, was sickened by it, wanted to leave Grover's Mill behind, but Ruthie's father insisted on remaining in town. He said that things would get better, and so I stayed as well. Ruthie's father was named Nathan, and he was a widower, an accomplished surgeon, and I had found it shocking to learn that a man who had helped to save the lives of so many invasion victims was being terrorized almost nightly by supporters of the Purity Movement. They claimed that they were defending the American Way of Life. If this was America, I wondered if Mars might be better.

We explored the rest of the farm, spoke about us, our mutual love, avoided talk about the grim world. We found joy in the rubble, and it was an odd thing, this juxtaposition between our feelings of destruction and renewal, and I wondered if it was because we were angry at Grover's Mill, if we wanted to see the entire town obliterated. The rubble reminded us of our beginnings as well. Ruthie's father saved my life. He found me lying on a downtown walk, gasping for breath as a cloud of greasy Martian smoke floated through the air. He covered his mouth, moved into the cloud, pulled me away, offered me life-giving breath from his own mouth. It was something I had never seen before, "resuscitation," he called it, and he told me that it was simple, a technique that every person could learn. The doctor's house was located a mile from the Wilmot farm, yet it had been overlooked by the Martians (another reason why some had accused him of having Martian blood), and the doctor was good enough to let me recover in his home. That was where I met Ruthie, and I believe that I fell in love with her the moment I set eyes on her.

We sat on the rim of the crater until the sun set, then watched the stars, in silence, for a long while. A meteor flashed across the sky, and I made a wish upon it, wondered if Ruthie had done the same. I saw her lips moving, her eyes closed, and then I knew that she, too, was praying that the arc of light had been a meteor, and nothing more.

I returned home and found a human skeleton hanging from the colonnade over my front porch. The morning light played upon bare bone, glowing yellow-red, deep shadows shrouded empty eye sockets. It was a teaching skeleton, I assumed, not the remains of an invasion victim, although to me, it was just as terrifying. This was a sign, a warning, similar in nature those which Ruthie and her father had been tormented with. Last week, Ruthie had found a human skull in her garden, in the midst of her poisoned roses. It was a symbol of the invasion, a way of saying that she was responsible. I had always worried about Ruthie, had felt angry, frightened, disgusted every time she was terrorized, but until that moment, I had never been threatened directly.

"Are you afraid?"

A Forager had spoken to me, and I had not been

aware of his presence until I turned and saw him standing a few feet away. His appearance shocked mc, and I wondered if he was the same Forager I had seen at the Wilmot farm. "Are *you* responsible for this?" I heard anger in my voice, which surprised me, because I felt only fear, felt violated by that swaying skeleton.

"No. I didn't do that. I'm a friend."

I laughed, and again, my reaction surprised me. My emotions were boiling over. "Go away. You won't find any cylinders here. No heat rays." I thought about the brooch I had given Ruthie, and it occurred to me that he might have been there to sell me Martian goods. He was just as young as the Forager I had seen at the Wilmot farm, just as frail, and I found myself feeling sorry for him. I had heard that many Foragers were orphans, children of victims who roamed the streets after the invasion without direction. "Whatever you want, I'm not interested." I stared at him and found no reaction in those dark eyes of his. "Do you know who hung that skeleton?"

"Yes." He waited.

"Tell me." I paused. "Please."

"They know about the baby."

"What are you talking about?"

The Forager smiled. His expression looked maniacal rather than friendly. "Maybe she didn't tell you."

"What? Stop playing with me." I grew more terrified, weak, as I thought about Ruthie. "Tell me."

"Your girl. The Martian—"

"What did you say?" I balled my fists, felt anger flush my cheeks.

The Forager backed up. His smile faded. "It's okay. We know about you. The baby will be half Martian. The first one—"

I lost control, hit him in the face. "I'm sorry," I said, and I watched him fall to the ground. I am thirty-two years old, and the Forager was easily half my age, half my weight. Hitting him had been an act of cowardice, of uncontrolled anger. I dropped to my knees, held my stomach, felt as though I was about to vomit. *Please, God, no,* I thought, *if Ruthie is pregnant . . .*

Tears stained with Martian makeup ran down the Forager's cheeks. He stood, looked at me, said "They know already. *Everybody knows already.*"

I looked at the skeleton again, and then I became more frightened as I thought about Ruthie's safety, about what the Purity Movement might do if they found out about our relationship, our *physical* relationship. Two minutes later, I was in my automobile, heading for Ruthie's home.

There were no skeletons on her porch, no skulls in the roses. When I arrived at Ruthie's home, Nathan was standing near the garden in his bathrobe. It seemed as though he was waiting for me. I once informed Ruthie that I wanted to tell her father about our mutual love, but Ruthie refused, told me that it would jeopardize our relationship. I said that she was wrong, and then all she told me was "I know my father better than you do," and that was it.

"Hello," I said, and I realized only then that my early morning appearance must have seemed odd.

"No bones."

"What?"

"There aren't any bones here. I never know what I'm going to find."

I noted that his demeanor seemed strange. He was unusually cheerful, though I felt as though he was masking some great pain, that he was a man who had secrets. Ruthie had told me that her mother had died at a young age, that Nathan had felt guilty for not being able to stop the cancer which eventually consumed her. "I'm sorry." I felt stupid.

"Not your fault." Nathan looked at me suspiciously. "How are *you* doing?"

"Fine. Just wanted to make sure everything was going well." I stared at his house, noted that everything looked in order. "Just passing by."

"You're up early." He put his hand on my shoulder, squeezed it in a friendly manner, said, "Are you going to celebrate the invasion?"

I looked into his eyes, at his hair which had gone gray during the last year. "It's nothing that *should* be celebrated." Something was wrong. I felt a remarkable tension between us.

He took his hand from my shoulder, said nothing.

I wondered if Ruthie had made it home before her father awoke. We had stayed at the Wilmot farm until an hour before dawn. I knew that Nathan would worry if Ruthie was gone for the entire night, and when I asked her about it, she said that she had lied to him. She had told her father that she was planning to walk into town in order to see the *The Thief of Baghdad* at the Metropolis, that she was meeting a friend, that she wanted to stay at her friend's house after the movie. I didn't believe that Ruthie had lied to her father. She simply wasn't good at it, hated the idea of lying, although I wondered why she would lie to me. The Metropolis hadn't admitted Negroes in months. Nathan knew that, so did I. If she had lied to her father, it was a very poor lie, one which he would have seen through. It occurred to me then that he had found out about our meeting, that he had known about our relationship for some time.

Ruthie's father moved closer, and to my astonishment, I smelled alcohol on his breath. "Be here tonight," he said.

"What?"

"Be here tonight." He backed up, smiled. "Don't you remember? The president will be speaking tonight. I thought that you might come and listen to the radio with us."

I had forgotten about Roosevelt's fireside chat. This evening, it would be devoted to the victims of the invasion. I had heard a rumor that the president had planned a visit to Grover's Mill today, the first anniversary of the Martian invasion, but it was canceled due to his declining health. "I'll be here," I said, and I felt uneasy. I watched Ruthie's father go back into his house, got into my automobile, and drove away.

The thought of Ruthie's pregnancy terrified me.

Flags flew at half-mast. As I drove through town, men hung black crepe from window ledges. Large signs bearing the message "We Shall Never Forget" had been placed within store display windows. I had grown accustomed to that message. It was everywhere, even in the pages of *Collier's* and the *Saturday Evening Post,* alongside the redesigned blue eagle of the new NRA. All businesses were closed for the day in honor of those who had lost their lives during the invasion, and as I looked at those motionless flags hanging in the still morning air, I felt as though I was driving through a tomb.

After I returned home, I walked around the house, then went inside. I expected to find something out of order, a broken window pane, mud tracked on the floor, but everything seemed right with the exception of the skeleton on the front porch. Exhaustion weighed me down, so I cut the skeleton down, threw it in the garbage, washed, went to bed. I doubted that I could sleep. Thoughts of Ruthie's safety, of my own, disturbed me, made me nervous and frightened, yet I fell asleep in moments, and did not wake until dusk.

President Roosevelt's speech would commence at seven o'clock, and I arrived at Ruthie's home by six. Nathan was civil, and when I arrived, a place had been set for me at the dinner table. We ate shortly after I arrived so that we would finish in time to sit by the radio and listen to the entire speech. Ruthie prepared a wonderful dinner, tender chicken with boiled potatoes, but for the most part, we ate in silence. I complimented Ruthie on her cooking, she smiled, nodded, her father ate, never spoke, rarely looked at either one of us. Ruthie and I were left alone in the kitchen as I helped her with the dishes, and I decided to move beyond the polite conversation which had held me back during the course of the evening.

"Something is bothering you," I said.

"No. It's nothing." Ruthie forced a smile.

"I need to know."

"Know what?"

I was growing tired of her polite banter, knew that she was holding something back. "Somebody threatened me yesterday." I hadn't intended to tell Ruthie about the skeleton, knew that it would worry her, but I was tired of deception.

Ruthie's smile faded. She put down the dish she was washing, turned off the water. "What are you talking about?"

"After we left the farm, I went home and found a skeleton hanging over my front porch." I looked into her eyes, saw that she was frightened. "I'm sorry. I shouldn't have told you."

"You don't have to protect me. I've seen so much of that. More than you. You're a white man . . ." She stopped herself, then said "Was anybody waiting for you? Did they hurt you?"

I felt angry, insulted. "Negroes aren't the only people who are threatened." We stared at one another, embraced, apologized for our comments. "It's been hard," I said.

"For both of us."

"Nobody threatened me."

"What?"

"When I came home. I found the skeleton, but nobody threatened me. There was a Forager . . ." I regretted bringing him up.

"What did *he* want. Do you think that he hung the skeleton? My God, what if they know about us? What if he hung the skeleton in order to threaten us both?"

"The thought hadn't occurred to me." I lied. "I imagine that somebody targeted my house by mistake." I wanted to tell her about my conversation with the Forager, ask her if she was pregnant, but I couldn't do it. We held each other until seven o'clock approached, then moved from the kitchen to the sitting room where the radio was located. Ruthie's father was standing outside the kitchen, and I knew that he had been listening to our conversation.

At that point, I no longer cared.

It was a nice Zenith floor radio, inlaid with burled wood, with a green eye which had little dark bands around a silver iris which grew larger or smaller according to the strength of the station. It reminded me of a Martian Crawler, of the hooded, green-eyed heat ray assemblies which had snaked up from the weird, shelled machines. Ruthie and I sat on the floor like children, waited for the radio to warm up, while Nathan watched and listened from an overstuffed sofa on the other side of the room. I tuned the radio dial, and after we listened to an advertisement for Barbasol and a lengthy introduction to the president's fireside chat, we heard Roosevelt's familiar voice.

"On October Thirtieth, Nineteen-Hundred and Thirty-Nine, forces from the Planet Mars did willfully, and with malice, attack the United States of America. It is a day which shall not be forgotten . . ."

As I listened to the president's speech, I wondered

how different things might have turned out if the Martians had invaded Germany rather than the East Coast of the United States, if the bacteria hadn't done them in, if the invasion had taken place on a world-wide scale. I wondered if they had touched down in Grover's Mill by chance, or if they intended to weaken the United States on the eve of another Great War.

". . . nameless, unreasoning, unjustified terror. We shall not fear . . ."

Ruthie stared at the radio dial, listened to the president's words as static cut in and out, and then she looked at me with tears in her eyes, took my hand as Nathan watched.

We heard something hit the roof. Nathan stood, moved toward a window. Ruthie and I followed, and as we stood before the window, we watched firelight play upon their hoods and robes. A dozen people stood near the house, torches in hand. Balls of flame arched across the night sky as a few of the men threw torches toward the house. One landed on the porch. Another thudded down the roof.

We stood, stared, calmly walked toward the back door. It was an odd reaction, completely logical, void of emotion. We might have screamed, I thought, tried to hide. Ruthie once told me that her father disliked guns, that he had been physically threatened so often that he would die rather than inflict violence upon another. We opened the back door, walked out, calm, orderly, accepting of fate.

They waited, rifles in hand, and we watched as one of them gestured with his weapon, told us with that long, dark barrel, that we should move to the front of the house. We obeyed, said nothing, and as we walked, we joined hands.

They surrounded us on the lawn, and under the smoky flames I looked at Ruthie's ruined garden, at their robes, and then I closed my eyes, tilted my head back. When I opened my eyes again, I saw the meteors. They streaked across the night sky, dozens of them, and I found myself smiling. I looked at Nathan and Ruthie, saw that they had followed my gaze, that they were smiling as well. We watched as a fireball arched across the sky, brilliant, sharp against the darkness, and with a blue flash it struck no more than five miles away, somewhere, I imagined, beyond the Wilmot farm. If these people were going to kill us, then that was how it would be. The Martians would kill them in time, complete their task, wipe Grover's Mill from the map. There was an odd, perverted justice to it. Nathan released my hand, pointed toward the sky, said, "See that one? That orange speck near that group of stars? That's *Mars*."

I doubted that the star or planet that Nathan pointed to was Mars, didn't remember whether the planet was visible during this time of the year, but it didn't matter. Any one of those lights in the sky might have been Mars, but they all meant nothing to me. Grover's Mill had become Mars for us.

They lowered their rifles, moved toward their trucks and cars, then one of them stopped, turned, removed his hood. His sweaty skin seemed to change color under his sputtering torch, and then I saw the gummy streams of makeup which ran from the corners of his eyes and mouth. The rest of them removed their hoods then, and I wondered how a real Martian would respond to those painted Martian faces of theirs, if they would think twice before burning those robed men to cinders. I doubted it. Orson Welles had told us that "intellect, cool and unsympathetic, regarded this Earth with envious eyes . . ." They drove away, toward the dull blue glow in the distance, and I knew that those men would not have a chance.

My mind filled with questions. I had assumed that the hooded men had been members of the Purity Movement, but as I thought about their faces, I wondered if they represented some odd faction of the Foragers, if they had not intended to kill us all along. I felt Nathan's hand upon my shoulder, Ruthie's arm around my waist, and my questions melted away. We turned, watched the house as fire licked through shattered windows, as the porch collapsed, as the second story spilled into the first. Sirens blared in the distance, toward that odd glow, and the house was left to burn. We made no attempt to save anything, and Nathan smiled as he watched, and I could feel his freedom. Ruthie and her father would leave now. Their was nothing left to hold them to Grover's Mill, and I would go with them.

I handed Nathan the keys to my Plymouth, then Ruthie and I sat in the back seat as Nathan drove away, leaving the burning house behind. We looked through the windows, watched as fireballs rained through the darkness, heard the distant hum of a heat ray. None of us said anything, and I wondered if Nathan had a destination in mind. It didn't matter. Ruthie slid across the seat, moved close, placed my hand over her stomach. I broke the silence, said, "Will it be—"

"A Martian?" Ruthie hugged me.

"Of course." I kissed her, said, "We're all Martians," and we drove through the night of the new world.